She Is Fasting

The Exclusive Women's Fasting Guide with 1000 Days of Fasting Recipes and 4 Fasting Meal Plans.

Dr Teresa Hill

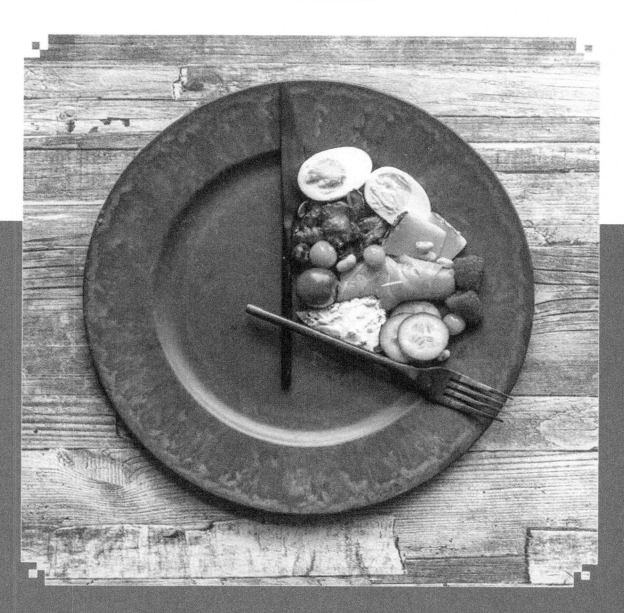

Editor: AALIYAH LYONS

Interior Design: BROOKE WHITE

Cover Art: DANIELLE REES

Food stylist: SIENNA ADAMS

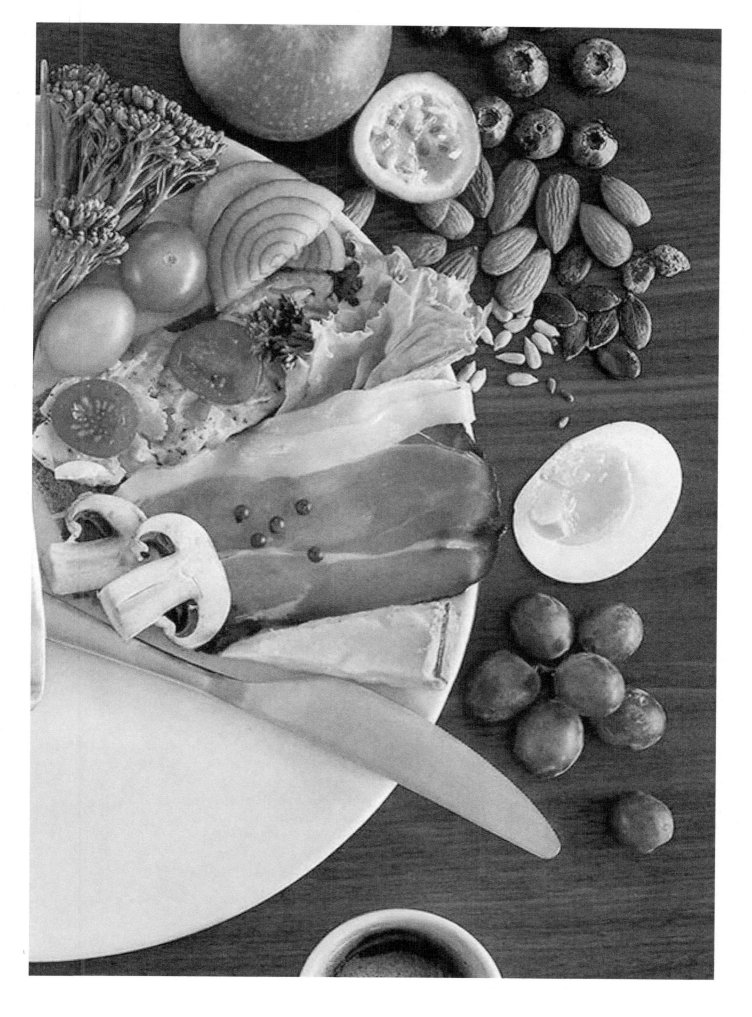

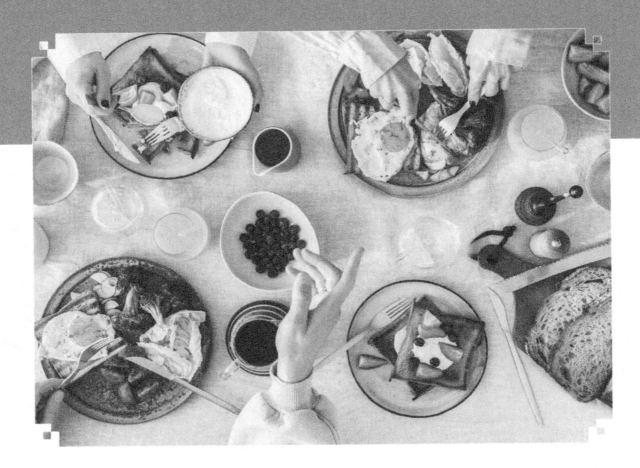

Table Of Contents

Introduction

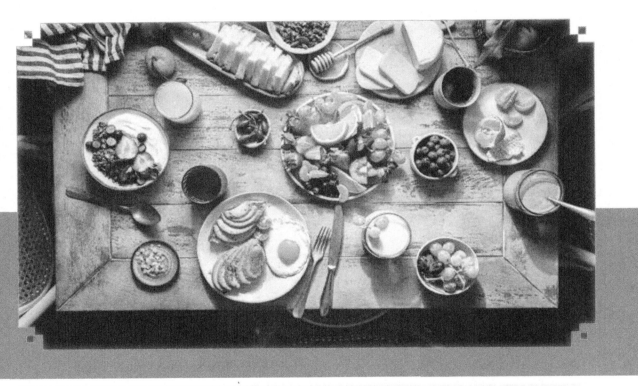

We women have never been in more need of a new method of being healthy. For the past few decades, the whole population has been facing numerous chronic conditions such as infertility, cancer, diabetes, cardiovascular disease, mood disorders, and different variants of chronic pains. However, women face most of these chronic conditions and still, both men and women are given the same solution. But the problem is there is a lot of difference in both male and female hormones so the one-size-fits-all solution rarely helps the hormonal needs which leaves the women feeling unheard, out of answer, and most importantly sick.

38 percent of American women have to go through hormone replacement therapy to deal with menopausal aftereffects. Even though this therapy is clinically proven to increase the risk of several types of cancer and cardiovascular disorders. And women are accepting the risks of cancer to deal with the hormonal issues. Another group of women choose different types of diets to lose weight but it is a temporary solution to a permanent problem. Along with that, the diet process they follow affects their mental and physical health in the long run. In simple words, these strict diet plans cause more harm than benefits.

Wondering what to do? What if I tell you that there is a fun and effective way to diet that helps to heal many chronic conditions? The method is called fasting. Fasting helps to lose weight, boosts mental health, improves organ function, and helps to gain a good metabolism. It allows you to lower the risk of chronic diseases by maintaining weight, maintaining energy levels, and sustaining bile health. FastingIn strict diet plans, there is a high chance of muscle mass loss but in IF the risk is lowered. Hunger and starvation are also managed in the case of IF. Along with all these benefits, IF helps to reduce belly fat which is a plus point for women who are worried about their belly fat.

Before getting into the details, let's learn how old age can be challenging for a woman. The hormones that keep our organs healthy and bodies active lower as we age. As a result, our organ system starts to fail, there is always a chance of a hormone being extremely low and another one being high. This inaccuracy causes the chronic disorders we face in today's world.

Our blood vessels lose their elasticity with age while the blood pressure increases. This is mainly done by stress and weight which are very sensitive factors in old age. The amount of blood pressure and stress increases with time and they lead to a major risk of cardiovascular diseases. Along with the stress, cholesterol buildup in the blood vessels also leads to heart-related disorders. It is a slow process but affects the body dangerously in the 50s. Blood sugar also starts to get unmanageable at this age and it can cause diabetes and related problems.

Besides all these conditions, our bones start to get more vulnerable. Lastly, hormonal imbalance is the biggest problem women face as they start to age. Hormonal imbalance affects the whole body and can lead to many problems. Because of this, women start experiencing problems like low energy levels, muscle stiffness, and bone weakness. We try to overcome these problems by eating high-calorie diets and instead of healing, we start to gain weight leaving us in misery. In simple words, eating a high-calorie diet is not the solution.

What you need as a woman is a diet plan that allows you to take nutrient-rich foods that are sufficient to meet your energy levels and keep your weight balanced. By a diet plan, I do not mean a typical plan that restricts you from eating everything and allows you to eat some specific dishes only. But fasting allows you to eat whatever you want but in a way that will keep your body healthy and your weight in check. Fasting is the best solution if you are struggling with weight management and dealing with post-menopausal hormonal imbalances. It will help you clear your endless tiredness and manage your blood sugar, cholesterol levels, and blood pressure at the same time. And last but not least, it will boost your mood as well as your mental health.

This "She is Fasting" book will help you discover the beauty of fasting and help you regain your strength. In this book, I will teach you the methods of fasting and provide you with customized effective meal plans. Besides this, we will also discuss the importance of working out while practicing fasting to get the best results. Most of the intermittent fast diet books only contain the basic methods and their application. But in this book, I am going to share my experience as a doctor and Woman. I also practice fasting so I am going to walk you through my personal experience and the peaks of success and failure. In my career, I have treated hundreds of patients who went through the same situation and I have seen a drastic change in both their physical and mental health.

In conclusion, I am going to teach you how to live a healthy life and how to Fast like a women!

Chapter 1

Stop Blaming Yourself, It is Not Your Fault

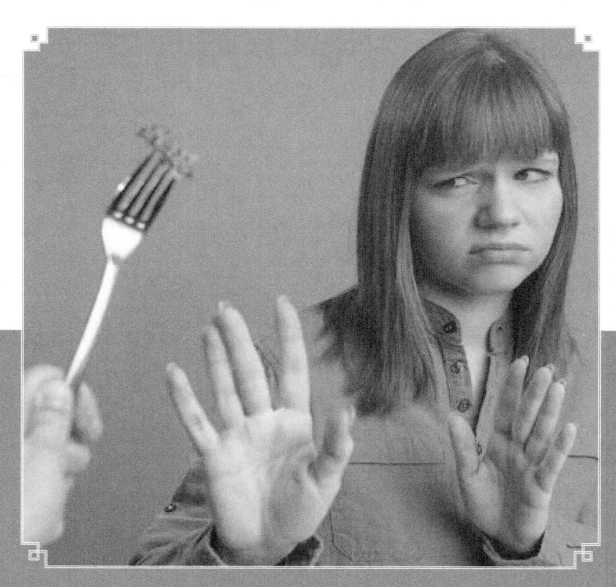

Stop blaming yourself, it is not your fault. The human body is a nearly perfect machine that contains more than 30 trillion cells. These cells work as a team to keep your body alive. Every cell in your body works a little factory that produces energy by burning ingredients like fat, metabolizing glucose, and manufacturing antioxidants in the body. These cells generate and store the energy and use it when your body needs it. Cells are aware of when you need energy and when you need to rest and they control the energy flow according to that. When we eat, our body breaks the food and allows the cells to take the nutrients and use them when needed. So what happens when you do not eat and cells do not receive a sufficient amount of nutrients? There is an alternative way to provide energy to your body. When your body senses that there is no food, the cells sense hormones open up their gates and let these hormones in. They can efficiently adapt to any physical, chemical, or emotional influence they face which is an amazing fact about your body.

However, to complete this process your body needs your support. The body's cells need certain nutrients to function properly. These nutrients include amino acids, good body fats, vitamins, and minerals. It is because the body cells take the reserved energy from these nutrients and supply it to your body. If there is nothing to use your cells will stop generating energy. Most of today's trendy diets are designed in a way that will finish your nutrients and this is why you feel tired. These quick diets work against your biological system and make it impossible to get a long-term result and on top of that lead you to many health issues. For this reason, in this chapter, I am going to explain the 5 ways diets have led you confused and tired. But the fun fact is you can correct them according to your body's needs. They are called the failed five and they include calorie restriction, poor food intake, cortisol surge, increasing toxic loads, and most importantly one-size-fits-all approaches. The most frustrating thing about these failures is that you see your friends go through the same diet and they get good results but it is the exact opposite for you. You get tired and gain weight instead of being healthy. If you ever approached a doctor after going through the same situation you know that doctors will tell you to lower your BMi and follow other one-size-fits-all methods. But you do not have to go through the same situation ever again.

Once I explain these 5 diet failures, you will understand what kind of health risks you were on. Understand that most of these diets are flawed. They disconnect your diet from your body and cause you to be frustrated and self-doubt and you blame yourself for the failure. To stop this madness, you have to understand how amazing the female body is and how to live it properly. But before that, you have to let go of the guilt and shame of not having a perfect body, a healthy life, and the diet failures you faced. There are too many women like you who blame themselves.

Everyone has battles. 80% of women face autoimmune conditions so there is nothing to be ashamed of, it is just natural. We are suffering as a collective group and these people are our mothers, sisters, grandmothers, friends, and other women. While the world needs women most we are not being able to give our all because of these hormonal conditions. And because of these problems, we are blaming ourselves, so before starting we need to accept the reality and be proud that we are contributing so much while we are fighting so many problems. So leave behind the negative thoughts and start to focus on keeping yourself as healthy as possible.

The Failed Five Methods

CALORIE-RESTRICTION DIETS

The biggest scam in the diet industry is counting your calories keeps you thin. This is a phrase that I want to permanently delete from your mind. All our life we have been taught that eating less and exercising more will help you live a healthy life. It is called the "calorie in, calorie out" theory and it is one of the hardest and longest-lasting ways to lose weight.

But isn't it the basic dieting theory, that you eat less and burn more to lose weight? Well, every time when you eat less and exercise more your body adapts the pattern and changes your metabolic set point. Metabolic set point means where the body maintains the weight in a more suitable range of calories. People used to believe that a set point is totally genetic. They believed that some people naturally have a high set point and some have a low set point. But modern science has proved it wrong and came up with a new theory. The truth is you train your set point with your own food intake. If you take less food and burn more it will lower your set point. This is how a low-calorie diet is ruining your health. For example imagine you continued to eat less and exercise more for 2 weeks, because of the diet your set point will fall and it will make it more difficult for you to continue the diet. And on top of that when you start to eat normally you gain more weight easily because you have lowered your set points! Isn't that scary?

But unfortunately, this is the very first diet we women try when we have to lose weight. This method brings some temporary results to keep you hooked. While you are getting some results, the brain will send hunger signals to your body and it will slow down your metabolism. Because of this reason, it is very hard to get permanent results from a low-calorie diet.

You might still wonder if it is true or not because you have been following this your whole life. So let's take a look at some case studies to clear your confusion. In the 1960s there was an experiment called the Minnesota starvation experiment. This is still one of the best and most accurate experiments done on a low-calorie diet. It shows how the diet affects your physical and mental health. For 13 months 36 men were progressively given lower amounts of foods until a 1500 calorie diet. While examining the subjects, there are several dramatic changes found in their physician and mental health. First, they started to get desperate at the thought of food until they could focus on their daily tasks. Following this reason, they became anxious and depressed and they started to become unsocial. Doesn't it seem like your last diet? But the worst was yet to come, when the experiment ended and they started eating normally they still faced mental health issues. And because of their low set points, they gained an extra 10 percent of the weight they started with.

If a diet is both mentally and physically threatening, you do not have to follow it. There is nothing more important than your health

POOR FOOD INTAKE

As people started to get more health conscious, they declared a war on fat. People were concerned that fat leads to cardiovascular diseases, and for that reason, we were instructed to stay away from every kind of fat. As everyone started to avoid foods that contained fat, food manufacturers were pressured to manufacture fat-free food. However, the food companies came up with another alternative. Instead of fat, they started using sugar and more flavorful ingredients. Because of the sugar intake, the obesity rate touched the roof. In the 1960's there was a survey where 14 out of 100 Americans were considered fat. In today's time, it has increased to 40 percent and if this goes on, the rate might increase to 50%.

In simple words today food companies are removing the fat from foods and replacing it with sugar. This is the reason you should not buy fat-free labeled foods because they are filled with sugar. Aside from sugar, there are also many flavors added, and both of them cause you to gain weight faster than fat could. This could be the end of the problem but no, all the processes you see in the market are causing you to lose in your diet game. There are many ultra-processed foods highly recommended in diets, which cause your body to become insulin resistant.

So what is insulin resistance? All their processed food causes your cells to change their nature and they do not use insulin as a hormone to collect sugar from your food. When the cells can not use sugar to make fuel, it stores the sugar as fat in your body and you feel weak. This condition causes many fatal metabolic syndromes that include high blood pressure, obesity, high blood triglycerides, low levels of HDL cholesterol, and most importantly high blood sugar. As you can see nearly everyone around us has some of these metabolic syndromes, know that we are collectively suffering.

So how does insulin work in your body? Insulin is basically a sugar-storing hormone. This hormone is released from the pancreas and its job is to escort the sugar from food to body cells. Insulin supply from the pancreas depends on how much sugar you are eating.

If a constant influx of insulin keeps hitting the receptors, the cell gates will become resistant to insulin. Which means the cells will eventually become numb to insulin. Once the cells become numb to insulin, both the sugar and insulin will be stored in your body as fat and push you towards greater diseases.

SPIKING CORTISOL SURGES

Cortisol is a great enemy to your diet. The fact is, you can not be stressed and build your health at the same time. So let's see how cortisol works and why it stops you from building health. Cortisol is spiked when your brain thinks you are under stress. For example, take one of the low-calorie diets you have tried earlier. Low-calorie diets often create stress, and the stress spikes the cortisol level. What happens is that when you eat less and work more, you feel irritated and hungry. It creates a fight-or-flight reaction in your brain and it responds by releasing cortisol into the bloodstream, to fight the crisis. In this situation, your body stops digestion, and fat burning and simply raises your glucose levels. When the glucose level rises, your pancreas releases insulin. The insulin floods your body cells and creates an imbalance. The worst part is all of this happens while you are not eating and still on your low-calorie diet.

Any diet that keeps you irritated and hungry will keep the cortisol level high and impact your dieting results. However, cortisol spikes don't happen with regular stress like work overloads, arguments with people, and other similar stuff. It only spikes while you are on a diet that does not fit your lifestyle. This can also happen when you workout too much and the body releases a ton of glucose to keep you working. The worst thing about cortisol spikes is you do not realize when it is happening. There are people who are dieting for a long time and building a constant flow of cortisol spikes that will eventually destroy their health. Cortisol is not mentioned in most diets but it has many side effects that can affect your goal of having a healthy body.

It is not important that you have to diet to have constant cortisol spikes. Day-to-day stress buildup can create a fight-or-flight simulation in your brain and it will spike a cortisol spike in your blood. And talking about a woman's body is way more sensitive to stress compared to a man's body. We are biologically designed to have hormonal imbalances when in stress. Women face more cortisol spikes compared to men and it often causes our sex hormones to drop and rise in insulin. If it keeps happening, no matter how long you have been dieting, or how long you work out, your body will face the consequences and you won't get the results.

Most diets do not keep the cortisol in check and this is how these diets have been failing you for years.

EXPOSURE TO TOXIC INGREDIENTS

Along with food, we intake some toxic ingredients as well. These are the toxic chemicals that are used in food to make it look more attractive and taste better. Toxins can make you fat. Toxins are so dangerous for your health that there is a category called obesogens. When these toxins enter your body, your body can not break them so it stores them as fat. You might wonder why the body does that. Well, the answer is your system stores them as fat so the chemicals do not harm any other organs in your body. This is a wonderful system our body creates for the long-term survival of your body.

The list of obesogenic chemicals is very long. However, these are the 5 worst kinds of obesogenic chemicals for your body: Phthalates, BPA plastic, atrazine, perfluorooctanoic acid (PFOA), and organotins. These chemicals have their presence in our daily essentials such as food, water, cleaning products, clothes, books, beauty products, and more. Monosodium glutamate and soy protein isolates are the most found obesogens in our foods. You can commonly find them in weight-loss shakes and related products. These chemicals work like insulin which blocks your cell receptors and makes it harder for the hormones to enter the cell gates. The rise of these chemicals can stop the thyroid hormones and insulin from entering your body cells which can lead to more weight gain, erratic mental health, and fatigue.

Avoiding and detoxing these chemicals can save your body from several health threats including, thyroid problems, weight loss resistance, and autoimmune conditions. The food companies will fool you with ingredient lists like all-natural, keto-friendly but do not be fooled. Check the packaging carefully and avoid all kinds of harmful chemicals. Not only that they will stop you from gaining a healthy body but they will also push towards other risks.

ONE-SIZE-FITS-ALL APPROACHES

The biggest problem with our diet system is that we think everyone can follow the same diet. No, there is no single diet for everyone. Each human being has different features and for that reason, they have to follow a diet that suits them. We all go through different hormonal needs in our lives and the diet must fulfill the hormonal needs for having a healthy life. Each of your sex hormones has different food requirements. Take estrogen for example, it requires a low-carbohydrate diet, on the other hand, progesterone requires a high-carbohydrate diet. This is the reason why your diet should suit your hormonal situation as well. Do not be surprised if you are hearing it for the first time, because most diet books do not tell you about this. If you are a cycling woman, eating the same diet daily can benefit you at the beginning but at the end, it will work against your body. The diets you have tried your whole life might just be a one-size-fits-all type of diet that does not benefit you. But the exciting part about being a woman is you can adapt your diet to your menstrual cycle. This is a technique we should learn and modify our diet according to the menopausal cycle. This can prevent many major problems women face today like infertility, polycystic ovary, and breast cancer.

This one-size-fits-all approach does not only harm you physically. This has a very negative impact on your mental health as well. When everyone follows the same diet plan, they go through different phases and the outcome is also different. Instead of creating our way of beauty we compare ourselves to each other and try to get the same results. We women all follow the same diet and try to get the same body. But as you learned earlier everyone's body is different and each body has different needs. So all these one-size-fits-all approaches are useless at the end. Keep in mind that even though we live in the same female body, our bodies' needs are not the same. Especially for women, we are all on our hormonal journey, so what we need is a diet that matches our needs. You do not need a diet that your friend tried and got benefits from, but you need a diet that will help you become the best version of yourself.

Finding the perfect diet for your body is very important to live a healthy life. This might seem very hard to understand but

believe me, as you learn more about how to fast like a women you will find it easy. The more you learn about dieting, the more you understand that your body is working for you, not against you. All your life you might have believed that your body works against you, these one-size-fits-all approaches have got you thinking like it.

Once you understand how your body works, you will see how effortless and fun dieting can be. To understand what your body needs you have to notice many details about your body. As you dive deep into this book, you find all these details and learn how to choose a perfect diet for you. The beauty of dieting starts with an inward journey, you will learn that your body is designed to heal itself. When you customize your diet according to your body, this works like the magic you have been waiting for your whole life.

Just know that you are more powerful than you think. But to start the journey you have to make three perspective changes. The first thing you need to let go of is your past. Just forget how many times you have failed. The second thing you need to do is promise yourself that you will never fall into the traps of these 5 failed methods. The third thing is to work for the dream you have been dreaming of for years, a healthy life.

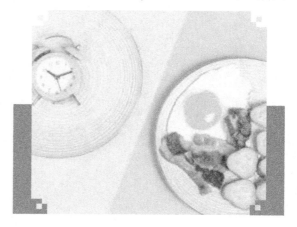

Chapter 2

What is Fasting and The History Behind Fasting

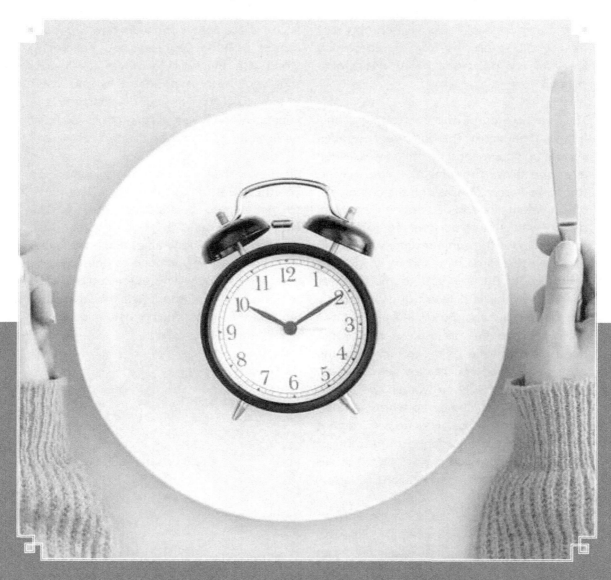

From the beginning of life, every living being depended on food. At the very beginning of the human race, our ancestors spent their whole lives looking for food just to survive. The only way to have food was hunting. This story is before even farming was invented so hunting was the only option. This is where the idea of fasting comes in. Fasting means not eating for a long time but eating whatever you like at a certain time. When our ancestors could hunt, they could eat, otherwise, they would have to fast without any kind of food. This cycle continued for hundreds of years and they survived while fasting. Fasting and hunting was the only way of life for our ancestors. The harsh life they lived has instilled a fasting instinct in our bodies. This is called the "thrifty gene", it explains that this genetic coding still exists in our body. It means when we do not follow what our ancestors used to do, we suffer from many chronic disorders. This is the reason why diabetes and obesity are major problems in today's world. Modern food companies have forced us to believe that we need to eat several times a day and keep our bellies full all the time. This is a war against our genetic code which has forced our body to become weaker and fall victim to numerous diseases.

Aside from ancient history, we can find fasting helpful in different cultures as well. In Muslim culture, Muslims fast for spiritual reasons. Muslims fasting during Ramadan is the biggest example of how easily and positively the human body can adapt to fasting. In Ramadan, Muslims fast for 30 days and some of the best fasting research is done during Ramadan. Aside from these, many more examples show that fasting was considered healthy and was practiced by a huge population. But are not we disobeying our ancestors' way of life and inviting more diseases? The answer is yes, we are forgetting the easiest and most effective way to live a healthy life. Fasting is effective for both men and women, but it can play a major role in maintaining the hormone levels of a woman. In this chapter, I am going to explain how fasting can turn on the healing switch inside you and what are the other benefits of fasting.

To understand everything about fasting, you need to learn a few things first. The first thing is that there are two fuel systems for your cells to complete their task one is sugar and another one is fat. The first fuel system is called the sugar burner energy system. It starts when you eat, the food you have eaten breaks down, and the sugar goes into the blood. When cells require energy, they use the sugar to complete their tasks and create more energy for your whole body. In the second method, things are quite different. It starts when you do not eat, it is called the fat-burner energy system or the ketogenic energy system.

It takes about 8 hours for your body to switch to the fat burner mode from the sugar burner energy system. This means you have to starve for 8 hours before your body switches to ketogenic mode. This is where fasting helps you, fasting for more than 8 hours which switches your energy system and burns extra fat from your body. Scientists today recommend fasting as the first line of treatment for many diseases including diabetes, obesity, cardiovascular diseases, cancer, and neurodegenerative brain conditions. It is proven that intermittent fasting has an anti-aging effect and can help you heal faster from surgery. Aside from these benefits, fasting can help us in many other ways with the metabolic which it causes. Some of the healing benefits include:

- Increased ketones
- Increased mitochondrial stress resistance
- Increased antioxidant defenses
- Increased autophagy
- Increased DNA repair
- Decreased glycogen
- Decreased insulin
- Decreased mTOR
- Decreased protein synthesis

One important fact about the human body is improving your metabolic health. To change metabolic health, you need to fix when you eat, not what you eat. In 2018 The Journal of Nutrition, Health & Aging published that obese people can dramatically get a metabolic improvement by fasting. They can eat whatever they want in 8-hour eating time and have to fast for the next 16 hours. Other similar studies also show the same result. This is sure that when you fast in this pattern, you will reduce your total body fat percentage, visceral fat. You can also gain lower blood pressure, decreased LDL cholesterol, and decreased hemoglobin A1c at the same time.

In today's world, we are eating low-quality food all day long while we are supposed to eat high-quality food at a certain time only. This has slowly changed our metabolic system and forced us to live a healthy life. If you are willing to change your metabolic health and live a healthy life this is the perfect time. Change your metabolic system by fasting and eating healthy foods. The best part about fasting is you do not need too many nutritious foods all the time and it is budget-friendly.

To understand how it works and the science behind it, you have to learn the major healing responses your body triggers when you are on an intermittent diet.

Increases Ketones

Ketones are an alternative fuel source from your liver that works when glucose is not enough. They are organic compounds that the liver produces when your blood sugar drops. This helps you burn the stored fat in your body. Having a low level of ketone surge in your body is a good sign. They are reparative which means they can go to certain tissues and help your body rebuild them. Ketones are good for your brain because they mainly focus on nervous tissue. They can improve your memory by regenerating the neurons that contain information. It is an effective and necessary compound for increasing focus and mental clarity. Aside from the brain, ketones are a good fuel for your cells' mitochondria.

Mitochondria's duty is to generate power for your cells and keep them working. With daily life stress and a bad eating habit, your mitochondria often can get tired. The ketones can reset them and give you consistent energy. The fun part is that ketone-generated energy is way different compared to glucose-generated energy. It will support you both mentally and physically. This wonder compound also helps your body to not feel hungry. When released from the liver, it goes up to your hypothalamus, turns off your hunger hormones, and also keeps you calm. Many people claim that they do not feel the hunger sensation when they fast, this is because of the ketone rush.

Increases Autophagy

Autophagy is a healing process that kicks in when you are fasting and your cells register dipping blood sugar. Your cells run this process to make them more resilient. The word autophagy means "self-eating". This healing process has 3 major benefits, detox, repair, and removal of diseased cells. Dr. Yoshinori Ohsumi, a Japanese scientist, came up with the brilliant concept of autophagy. He revealed that our cells get stronger in the absence of food. When you do not eat, cells start eating what is preserved inside the body. This is how autophagy detoxes your body by eating the harmful compounds stored in your body. No wonder why Dr. Yoshinori Ohsumi won the Nobel Prize in 2016 for physiology. This research was so important and popular, that many other researches were conducted for more information about autophagy.

This is a form of detox and for that reason, it is heavily praised in the fasting world. It removes the harmful compounds from the cells that were interrupting them. Your body goes through a major cell reboot and many people feel younger after going through the autophagy process.

A study in 2020 shows that autophagy is highly effective in fighting the COVID-19 virus. As viruses do not own an energy system, they depend on the prey's body cells. If the body is in sugar-burning mode, viruses can take energy from there and work. But if your body is in an autophagy state, viruses can not take energy and replicate.

Autophagy is also able to remove the old and worn-out cells from your body. As every cell works as a factory, they get old and ineffective with thyme. When you force your body to go into the autophagy mode your cells start eating the unnecessary parts and remove the malfunctioning cells.

The only limitation of autophagy is it can only remove organic compounds from your cells. Synthetic and man-made chemicals like plastic, perfluoroalkyl, and poly-fluoroalkyl can not be removed by the autophagy

process. This can not also recycle heavy materials like lead and mercury. Natural heavy materials like them can damage your brain and hormonal system as well as your mitochondria. Autophagy has a special feature known as apoptosis. In this process, rogue cells that often cause problems in your system are killed. These cells can also turn into cancer cells so killing them is the best step for long-term health. Along with these benefits, autophagy contains the power of healing mitochondria, this is also known as lithography and this can save you from muscle weakness, hearing, vision problems, and many other problems we women face today.

Growth Hormone Rise

Growth hormone is considered the fountain of youth. This hormone runs in your veins when you are a child but as you age, the production of growth hormone is lowered. Growth hormone flow stays at its peak during puberty and lasts until 30 years old. And right after growth hormone starts to fade from your body, your body starts aging. For this reason, people face many aging issues after 30 and start to have mental and physical changes. Growth hormone plays a vital role in burning fat. This also helps in muscle building, this is the reason young people can gain better health by exercising. Another thing about growth hormone is it is essential for healthy brain development. As a teenager, you learn many things so this is where the growth hormone stays the most. As you have aged your need for learning has lowered so did your growth hormone.

But how about we want to raise the growth hormone in our body to burn fat, build muscles, and learn new things? Fasting can help you increase the growth hormone

release in your body. As you start fasting, your body will release growth hormones depending on the length of your fast.
Resets dopamine pathways

Have you noticed how food excites you? Well, this is because of dopamine. Dopamine is a hormone that gives you a sense of pleasure and achievement. When you receive more dopamine daily, you can become a dopamine addict. Just like your cells get insulin resistant from too much insulin, dopamine overflow can affect your brain and keep you in a gloomy mood. There are several sources of dopamine like your Doordash guy came with a delivery, your phone's notification, and many other things. The one source that gives a consistent dopamine rush is food. Every Time you have a dopamine release, you will need more dopamine to feel good in the future.

Many people depend on food for dopamine. They believe that more eating will help them be happy, but in reality, the dopamine rush will slowly destroy your mental health and you will become overweight. As your dopamine receptors become resistant to it, it is very hard to reset this dopamine pathway. But the good news is dopamine pathways can be reset with different light fasts. Fasting not only helps you reset the dopamine level but it also makes your dopamine receptors more sensitive so you can feel much pleasure in less dopamine.

Improved Microbiome

We all know that the human body is full of bacteria. But did you know that the body contains 10 times more bacteria compared to human cells? All of these bacteria are not bad, some of them have positive and some have negative impacts on your cellular system. 90% of these bacteria live in your guts and others live all around your body. So what is the purpose of bacteria in our body? The main task in the human body is to pull vitamins and minerals out of your food. It makes neurotransmitters like serotonin, which break down estrogen. They also scan your cells for inflammation in case that needs to be lowered. These bacteria work hard to support your cells.

But we are constantly killing those bacteria in many methods. Foods, medicine, even the wifi in your house are killing the helpful microbes in your body. And the dangerous thing is taking a round of antibiotics can kill 90% of your gut microbes, can you imagine how much impact it will have on your cells? These microbes work super hard to support your cells and the instant death of so many microbes will change your delicate microbe balance. Having a microbe imbalance is risky, there are 2 very important microbes in your gut: Bacteroidetes and Firmicutes. An obese person has more firmicutes than Bacteroides, which causes the body to store calories as fat. On the other hand, if anyone has more Bacteroides compared to Firmicutes, they are more likely to stay healthy.

Microbes help you to complete many important tasks in your body. Weight loss, breaking down estrogen and neurotransmitter production are just some of those tasks. Microbes control everything from how hungry you are to the foods you crave. It is proven that people with more microbial diversity are less hungry and healthy. The best thing about fasting is it can bring back those microbes in your body. Fasting improves your microbial diversity, increases the production of bacteria that turn white fat into brown fat, pushes microbes away from the gut lining, and regenerates stem cells. These four factors can play a crucial role in your weight loss.

Prevents Cancer To Reoccur

A journal from the American Medical Association in 2016 released a study about cancer. More than 2000 women between the ages of 27-70 were diagnosed with breast cancer. After analyzing this group an amazing fact about fasting was discovered. It shows that women who fasted for more than 13 hours a day, had 64 percent less chance of reccour breast cancer. So how does it work? Fasting significantly decreases the hemoglobin A1c and c-reactive protein. One works as an indicator of glucose in blood and the other indicates inflammation. There are very few drugs that can offer this kind of result. Fasting not only stops cancer from reccour but it also prevents cancer in the first place. And the wonderful news is it can prevent many other types of cancer aside from breast cancer.

All these amazing facts must have got you excited! You have a deeper knowledge of fasting now and in the next part, you are going to learn different types of dieting and choose the best for you. So without any delay, let's learn more about fasting!

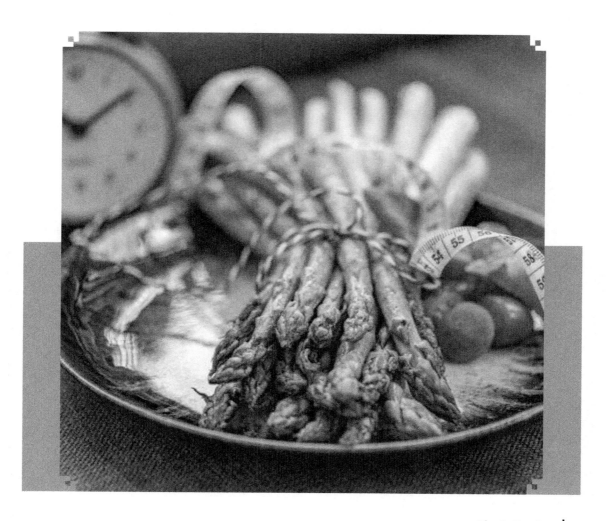

Chapter 3

Six Different Types of Fasts

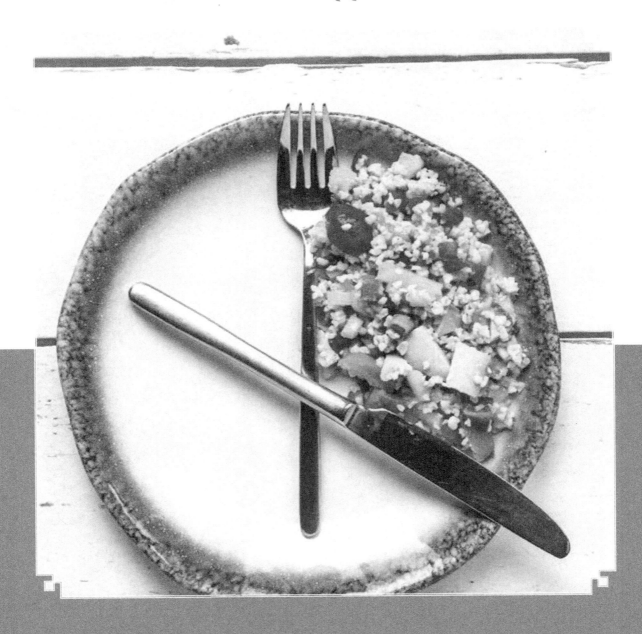

The word fasting is quick and easy, but there are different types of fasting to achieve your specific goals. The key difference between each fast is their lime length, each fast brings different results. So let's break down these six fasts and choose the best fast for you!

1. Intermittent fasting: 12–16 hours
2. Autophagy fasting: starts at 17 hours
3. Gut-reset fast: 24 hours
4. Fat-burner fast: 36 hours
5. Dopamine-reset fast: 48 hours
6. Immune-reset fast: more than 72 hours

Intermittent Fasting (12–16 Hours)

Intermittent fasting is the most popular type of fasting. Most people follow this fasting and do not eat for 12-16 hours a day. To understand intermittent fasting from the core you have to go through a 24 hours cycle. For example, let's say you finished your dinner at 7 and you stopped eating or drinking anything from that time. You go to bed and after waking up, you take your breakfast at 10 a.m. so that is logically 15 hours of fasting. In the meantime, your liver will switch and start making ketones. Ketone production starts when your body goes without food for 8 hours. And when the fast is between 12-15 hours, your body switches to ketogen mode and it makes energy by burning fat.

At first, ketones flow in your brain and slowly reach your brain, they simply turn off your hunger sensation and boost your physical and mental energy. The body cells go into an autophagy state and start repairing, regenerating, and detoxing themselves. As you are fasting there is a shortage of glucose in your body, your liver senses the absence and breaks down fat to supply glycogen and insulin. Once you start fasting regularly, you will see a huge change in your metabolic system. It will help you control your blood pressure, hemoglobin, c-reactive protein, glucose, and insulin. The microbes in our gut will also regrow because fasting kills the bad bacteria. It will help you improve your microbial makeup and allow your body to more more mood-fixing neurotransmitters. Increasing these neurotransmitters is crucial for your mental health.

Intermittent fasting is one of the easiest fasts so take it as a path to enter fasting. It is easy to do and maintain with your daily tasks. Intermittent fasting is perfect for people who feel weight-loss resistant in their body, experience brain fog, and feel tired all the time. Intermittent fasting burns energy from stored fat instead of sugar. This is a hugely beneficial step you can take for your body.

Fasting might seem like hard work at first, but if you follow some simple steps it is easy to do. If you are fasting you can follow a few steps to make it effortless and helpful for you. Eat your meals in an 8 to 10-hour meal period and leave the rest hours for fasting. To begin the process, delay your breakfast 1 hour. Continue the same process for a week and again push your breakfast time to an hour. Keep this routine until you can comfortably fast for 14 hours. You can also delay your dinner but eating too late and going to bed instantly will affect your weight loss process. So let's see how it will help you lose weight, clear brain fog and restore energy.

WEIGHT LOSS

There are numerous ways to lose weight but intermittent fasting is the best. There is no doubt that it will help you lose weight and there are hundreds of women who have lost weight by this fasting. This process simply changes your metabolic system and goes to fat-burning mode. Fat is extremely hard to burn and because it will burn your fat you will lose weight quickly and in a healthier way.

BRAIN FOG

Brian's fogs are an irritating and distracting mental state. But once you start fasting it will feel like someone turned a switch in your brain and everything seems clear. You will be able to focus on tasks more attentively. This happens because of ketones, when you are fasting for 15 hours your liver generates ketones and they start working with your brain. Because of the ketone's ability to clear your brain, many people fast before tests, speech, or any activity that requires mental clarity.

RESTORE ENERGY

The energy we generally get comes from food. Different types of food deliver different types of energy, for example, if you take carbohydrates you will feel an energy bust but it will also instantly fade leaving you in a sleepy situation. On the other hand, if you take a protein-focused meal, you might not feel an energy bust but it will keep you going at a certain level.

But, the thing about intermittent fasting is different. In this process, your body starts burning fat to provide you with energy. This ketone energy is different from other sources. You will feel it suddenly and it will keep you energetic for a long time without any crashes.

Autophagy Fasting (17-72 Hours)

Autophagy is just another fasting process that requires more time compared to intermittent fasting. Autophagy kicks in when you are fasting for 17 hours and it reaches its peak at 72 hours. Many benefits of autophagy fasting are different from intermittent fasting. Autophagy is perfect for people who are looking to detox,

improve their immune system, improve their brain function, and balance their important sex hormones.

DETOXIFICATION

Autophagy is a perfect tool for detoxing your cells. It works great when your cells go through the pressure and they are worn out. For example, you can try autophagy after your vacation where you are running around, exploring new places, and trying new foods that harm your system a bit. This is the perfect time to start autophagy. Another wonderful thing about autophagy is it can heal mitochondrial damage when there are too many toxins in your body.

INCREASE BRAIN FUNCTION

As we age, we start to feel confused and can not focus much. This is because our brain cells are aging too and some of the brain cells stopped working. Autophagy is a powerful weapon to increase your brain's functioning power. It can slow down your brain cells aging, enhance your mood, and improve memory cells in your brain. Whenever you feel unfocused and feel like forgetting everything, just start the autophagy fast and experience the wonder.

IMPROVE IMMUNE SYSTEM

Autophagy fast is a great way to improve your immune system. When you are on an autophagy diet, there is very little energy left in your cells. As bacteria need to feed on your energy, they are not that effective at the time. You can very easily avoid colds and related diseases with autophagy. And a fast that is longer than 17 hours will improve your immune system and help you stay strong.

BALANCE YOUR SEX HORMONES

At this time, every woman goes through some hormonal issues in life. Most of these problems occur because of sex-hormonal imbalance. Fasting during your perimenopause years like when you are trying to get pregnant can help. Studies show that the key cause of hormonal problems is dysfunctional autophagy. Autophagy fasting helps with menstruation and reduction in inflammation. Weight loss which is the cause of PCOS.

Gut-Reset Fast (24+ Hours)

If you are looking to heal your body from the core, gut reset fast is a perfect choice. In this process you have to fast for 24 hours or more, it supplies stem cells into your gut to heal itself. Our gut is often damaged because of the chemicals and medicine we take. This fasting can magically improve your gut health. Stem cells only produce in your body when you are fasting for more than 24 hours, it finds the worn-out cells and brings them back to life. Many people have to pay for the stem cells to be injected into their body, but why pay when you are getting the benefits just by fasting? When you fast for 24 hours, the microbes in your gut will help your immune system to make neurotransmitters that keep the brain happy, focused, and calm.

Gut reset fast is appropriate for healing antibiotic effects, intestinal bacterial overgrowth, and recovery from birth control.

HEALING ANTIBIOTIC EFFECTS

Our gut is full of bacteria and there are both good and bad bacteria in our body. But the problem is antibiotics not only kill the bad bacterias but it also kills the good bacterias as well. Taking a round of antibiotics can kill 90% of your bacteria. By fasting for 24 hours, you can heal the good bacteria in your body and bring your life back on track.

HELP TACKLE SMALL INTESTINAL

BACTERIAL OVERGROWTH

SIBO or small intestinal bacterial overgrowth is a condition where there is bacterial growth in your small intestine. It can cause you many problems like bloating. There are very few medicines for this cause although none of them work properly. However, fasting for 24 hours can kill the bacteria in your small intestine. As you fast for 24 hours, those bacteria have nothing to eat and they slowly get tired until their death.

RECOVERY FROM BIRTH CONTROL

Just like antibiotics, birth control pills create a microbial imbalance in your system. It also causes a leaky gut and creates a perfect environment for yeast to grow. When someone has a leaky guts they have a major risk of falling sick. A leaky gut is a condition where the tight junctions of the thin mucosal lining open up and many harmful objects can get into your blood. It creates a systemic inflammatory condition. The bad news is stop taking these pills won't help your gut but a 24-hour fasting can. This 24-hour diet is more helpful than other medications for curing leaky gut.

Fat-Burner Fast (36+ Hours)

Most people join fasting because of losing weight. It has gone to everyone's ears that fasting can play a very effective role in weight loss. The fat-burner fast is also very famous for the cause, it requires you to fast for 36 hours to burn your fat. Fat burner fast can help you decrease weight loss resistance, burn stored sugar, and reduce cholesterol levels.

DECREASE WEIGHT LOSS RESISTANCE

People are slowly becoming weight-loss resistant and the key reason for this is our diet. We are eating processed unhealthy food and for that reason, our body is resisting to lose weight. But this problem can be fixed with just 16 hours of intermittent fasting. But many people do not get the result from intermittent fasting, this is where the fat-burner fast comes in. This is a 36-hour fast that can help you lose weight magically. All those poor diets caused your body to store that extra sugar. It might be tough for you to fast for 36 hours but it comes in handy by practicing the 16 hours and 24-hour fasts.

BURN STORED SUGAR

People often face blood sugar imbalance while fasting. This is the natural way of releasing sugar in your body. This sugar is stored in your muscles, tissues, and liver. Most women do not permanently lose weight before this sugar-burning or releasing process. Fasting is the best possible way to do it. And if you want the process to be faster, insert 36-hour fasts in your routine and enjoy the magic.

REDUCE CHOLESTEROL LEVEL

Cholesterol level rises when your liver has been dealing with high influxes of sugar, toxins, and fats. The liver also makes ketones which can be jump-started with a 36-hour fast. As you diet regularly, you will see your cholesterol level reducing, and doing it regularly can help you reach your goal of a healthy body.

Immune-Reset Fast (72+ Hours)

The immune reset fast, also known as a three to five-day water diet, is very beneficial for health. To get the benefits of this fast you have to fast for 72 hours or more. But people who fast regularly like to stretch the time up to five days. The reason many people go up to 5 days is because after fasting 72 hours your body starts to generate stem cells that can find injured body parts and heal them. Fasting for 72 hours and not generating extra stem cells will be a loss, for that reason many people even extend it to 5 plus

days. These stem cells have amazing healing effects and they are helpful for many other reasons. As a doctor, I recommend it to people who are looking to solve a chronic condition, prevent chronic conditions, slow down the aging effect, and relieve pain.

EASE A CHRONIC CONDITION

This 72-hour fast is going to be hard for some people but it provides amazing outcomes. There was a test on patients going through chemotherapy and it has been proven that patients with cancer diagnosis can get help. It nourishes your immune system by removing ineffective white blood cells. This can be very helpful for someone who is being treated for cancer, type-2 diabetes, a frozen shoulder, etc.

PREVENT CHRONIC CONDITIONS

Practicing this three-day fast 2-3 times a year can be very helpful and it can help prevent cancer. We all have cancer cells inside us and a good immune system stops it from spreading. Trying this fast 2-3 times a year will kill those cells and give your body a healthy environment.

ANTI-AGING

72-hour fasts can help you stay younger. This is because a 72-hour fast generates stem cells and those cells can heal other cells. So whenever they're in your blood, they will detect the damaged parts and start healing them. If someone is looking for an anti-aging method, they can extend the 3-day fast to 5 or more days. This is an amazing way to slow your age and heal your organs.

After learning so many facts about fasting and its benefits, you must be motivated. You now understand the importance of fasting in a woman's life. In this "She is Fasting!" book I will explain more facts about fasting and help you find the perfect fast for you.

Chapter 4

Fast Like a Women

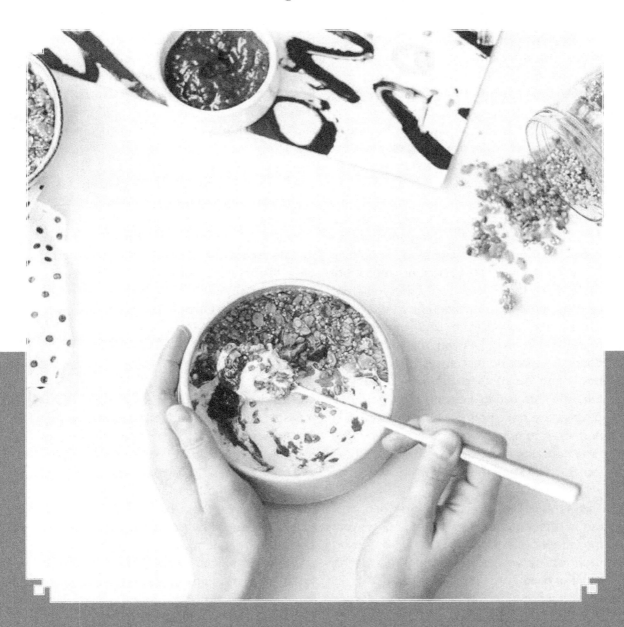

Fasting is an effortless exercise that will help you achieve your goals. Both male and female bodies are appropriate for fasting. But the twist is that the female body reacts differently from the male body when fasting. This is because of the hormonal difference between a male and a female. Even every woman can not fast the same way. I have seen many women who have benefited from fasting but after 6 months or a year of fasting, they encounter different symptoms such as anxiety, panic attacks, depression, and many others. You might wonder how this is possible, the answer is yes this is possible and this happens for a valid reason. The female body you and I live in is way more complex than you think. Because of the menstrual cycle, our bodies go through a rollercoaster of hormonal changes. The best way to fast is to sync your fasting habit with your menstrual situation.

I know it is still a bit confusing so let me explain it to you. The first thing you need to know as a girl is that your body is unique. Every woman has their unique menstrual cycle and the cycle can have different lengths. Most of the women have a 28-day cycle, some have shorter and some can go more than 30 days. As your menstrual cycle continues, your hormones rush through your body and maintain a consistent rise and fall. The interesting part is each hormone pushes the next hormone. This means if a hormone completes its tasks properly, the next hormones will also be able to do their job. But if one hormone lags, other hormones will also lag.

This is the reason why you should fast like a women and fast according to your menstrual cycle. In the next part, I am going to introduce you to the appropriate fasting cycle of a woman.

The Fasting Cycle of a Women

A woman's body is way complex you can imagine. For that reason, fasting for a woman is not only starving for 13 hours a day. Before fasting, we have to sort out all the hormones and fast according to our menstrual cycle. If our fast can't sync with the menstrual cycle, instead of having a healthy body you will become a mess. But if you fast according to your menstrual cycle, you will get amazing results. Syncing your fast cycle with the menstrual cycle will balance your hormones, charge your cells with energy, and be the best fat burner option. But how to sync your cycles? Do not worry because I have created a map of the cycle according to different menstrual conditions.

The maps will help you follow different fasts to achieve the same goal. This fast suits your body and permanently removes the one-size-fits-all concept from your fasting routine. These plans are flexible and cover all of the important days for you. In the next part, you will learn how the fasting cycle works and the 3 types of fasting cycles.

How The Fasting Cycle Works

The fasting cycle plan is synced with your menstrual cycle to provide the best results. The first thing you need to know about the fasting cycle is it breaks down your menstrual cycle into three phases. These cycles are called the Energy Phase, the Transformation Phase, and the Care Phase. These are named after your moods influenced by hormones in the specific phase. Breaking it down to you, in the energy phase you can focus more and go for longer fasts. During the care phase, you are supposed to slow down and take care of yourself with healthy foods. In the transformation phase, you fast less compared to the power phase and let your body get ready for another energy phase.

Our fasting cycles are built around 30 days but every woman has a different period cycle. Some have 28 and some can go up to 32 days. To make it easier for you, our plan is designed in a way that everyone can follow. If you have a 28-day cycle, you have to follow the process until 28 days. Once your period starts you are one day one again and if you have a 32-day cycle follow a 30-day fast and stay in the care phase until your period starts again.

As I said earlier, there is no one-size-fits-all approach so follow the fasting and food suggestions but experiment with each option. It will help you find the best option for yourself. And if you are worried that you never tried to fast before, or have an irregular cycle, do not worry. In the next chapter, I will provide more information about fasting and it will help you to start fasting. Every process of how to fast like a women. This information will help you find out more about fasting and customize it your way. Trying new fasts can have magical changes in your body. But remember to do them the right way or else it can provide opposite results. Your body will get the best benefits once you find your fasting rhythm.

There are 3 fasting phases, 6 different fasting lengths, and 2 core eating styles you need to learn before fasting. So let's deep dive and learn all that information to get the best results of fasting.

The Energy Phase
Fasting length: 13-72 hours
Optional food style: ketobiotic
Focused hormone: Insulin and estrogen
Focused healing method: Autophagy and ketosis

In our fasting cycle energy phase is where you fast longer than 17 hours. This is called the energy phase because your body can take that much pressure. In your energy phase, you can maximize all the healing methods because your sex hormones stay low at this phase. In the menstrual cycle, there are only two times when your sex hormones stay low when you first start bleeding and after you ovulate. These are the days when you feel more emotionally stable and have more energy. At this time you are less hungry and have a great opportunity to fast longer.

In the first energy phase which is between 1-10 days, your body produces estrogen. Because the estrogen hormone is responsible for telling your ovaries to release the egg. For that reason, ovulation is impossible without estrogen. At the beginning of this phase, estrogen is produced slowly but as it gets closer to 10 days the estrogen production increases a lot. In this situation, if you are on a high-carbohydrate diet and eating six meals a day, it might be hard on your body. When you are high on carbohydrates, your insulin level rises and it can create a deficiency in your estrogen production. This was the short-term scenario but in the long term, it can lead to hyper-production of testosterone. Just know that when your insulin level rises, estrogen goes down.

The second energy phase which is between 16-19 days has a large impact on your hormonal production. At this point all the hormonal surges that occurred in the transformation phase start to come off. As the hormones stay very low in this state you might feel less motivated and have a shortage of energy and clarity. These 4 days can be proven very effective by fasting more than 17 hours. It will stimulate autophagy in your body and repair your gut, burn fat, and improve your dopamine pathways as well as reset your immune system.

For the healing process, you have to target autophagy and ketosis. fasts that are shorter than 17 hours improve your fat-burning capabilities. On the other hand, longer than 17 hours is more repair-focused. Autophagy targets certain areas in your body and heals those parts. The neurons in the hormonal control center in your brain can be helped by autophagy. It heals the neurons and provides them with important nutrients to be more precise in their work. To provide healthy and balanced hormones, your brain ovaries need to be healthy. Years of high insulin and toxic exposure might have affected these body parts but autophagy can help them work freely. This is similar to a sink that can get clogged with waste, the insulin and toxins can clog the cells of your brain and ovaries which can stop hormone production. Practicing autophagy will clear those clogs and help your cells to produce more hormones. When autophagy cleans your cells, the ketones produced by the kidney power your cells. This is a very important element for your mitochondria so they give their best. The autophagy and ketosis phase is a perfect healing combination for a healthy life and it makes the organs ready for the next phase of hormone production.

As for your food, I suggest eating foods that have low glucose and insulin production. By lowering your glucose intake, you can take the full advantage of xenobiotics. After fasting for 17 hours, try to break it with food that has good fat and salad.

The Transformation Phase (Days 11–15)
Fasting length: Less than 15 hours
Optional food style: hormone-feasting food
Focused hormone: estrogen, testosterone
Focused healing Organ: supporting a healthy gut and liver

This is the best part of this 30-day fasting cycle. In this phase, estrogen and testosterone stay at the peak and there is a mild surge of progesterone. All of these hormones are a perfect combination for making you happy and your best. During these 5 days, you are most fertile and ready to make a baby. The estrogen will spark your creativity, and add more glow and shine to your skin and hair. All of these hormonal synchronization might make you a bit talkative as well. With the estrogen boost, you can become an incredible multitasker.

During this time, you also get a good amount of testosterone and it fires up your libido and gives a boost of motivation. You can achieve many things you want like running a marathon, joining the gym, and other things that need a lot of motivation. In this phase, our main focus is to metabolize the hormones. Metabolizing hormones means breaking down your hormones in a more usable way and preparing those hormones for excretion. The liver and gut help you to metabolize the hormones and once they start working you will feel a hormonal boost in your body. Estrogen is very important for detoxification. When the estrogen is not properly broken down and excreted from your body, it will be stored in your tissues. Unmetabolized estrogen in your body can lead to danger, it causes weight gain and many hormonal cancers including breast cancer. It can lead to many other premenstrual symptoms like night sweats, breast tenderness, and moodiness. In this transformation state, you have to metabolize all the estrogen.

The best way to metabolize estrogen is to avoid long fasts and eat foods that nourish your liver and gut. Hormone-feasting foods can help in this case. They can improve bile production for breaking down fat and improve digestion. The most important thing about this phase is you can not fast longer than 15 hours. The toxins stored in your tissues need to be released before triggering autophagy. If you fast for 17 hours in this state it can create a detox reaction that can lead to nausea, brain fog, anxiety, muscle aches, and vomiting. So in this phase, fast for less than 15 hours, and eat hormone-feasting foods.

So now let's talk about our other targeted hormone testosterone. In this phase, you are supposed to get the largest testosterone surge. This is an amazing hormone for girls and it gives us motivation and fires up our libido. If you are not going through the same situation, it means you are low on testosterone. This is because food and fasting is not the most effective way of increasing testosterone. Instead, removing toxins and major stressors from your life are the most impactful steps you can take to balance your testosterone level. Try to avoid phthalates because they are highly dangerous for your testosterone production. However, this material is available in many regular-use products like plastic, and personal care products with high fragrances like shampoo, soap, and perfume. Avoiding phthalates is a smart move to increase your testosterone levels.

Stress can also play a big role in your testosterone imbalance. It can suppress the production of progesterone and testosterone which requires DHEA. cortisol also needs DHEA for production. When your body is stressed it will focus on making more cortisol instead of progesterone and testosterone. It will create a deficiency of these 2 hormones and you might feel less motivated during this time.

The care phase (Day 20–First Day of Your Period)
Fasting length: No fasting
Optional food style: hormone-feasting food
Focused hormone: cortisol, progesterone
Focused healing method: Reducing cortisol
This is the phase you should care about your body the most. However, stress in this state can bring out many hormonal consequences. Stress and lack of sleep destroyed a very important hormone known as progesterone. This hormone calms your body and tells your brain that everything is okay and in control. Just like the name of this phase, you have to take care of your body in this phase. There are a total of three ways to take care of yourself in this state. The first step is skipping fasting. You have to skip fasts because fasting can create small spikes in cortisol that can reduce the production of progesterone. Cortisol can also be raised by over-exercising and pushing your physical limits. In this phase, shift from hard workouts to effortless easy workouts like yoga, hiking, and long walks.

As you are not fasting in this phase, you have to eat more hormone-fasting foods. You can eat the same foods you ate for your liver and gut during the transformation phase. The fun fact about this phase is your body gets more insulin resistant because your body needs more glucose to make progesterone. Fasting and trying to start ketosis in your body can be proven destructive in this phase. This is because your body needs more carbohydrates at this time. The glucose will increase progesterone production and calm your body. Once the progesterone hits its peak, your periods will start and you will start the fasting cycle all over again.

Just remember to eat foods that help your body to create more progesterone such as Sweet potato, red potato, russet, and purple potato. Squashes such as spaghetti, butternut, and honey nuts. Citrus fruits such as lemons, limes, grapefruit, oranges, Pumpkin seeds, etc. This way the progesterone production will be very low and your PMS symptoms will be at their worst. You will start skipping periods and your uterus will be unable to hold a fertile egg as well.

Chapter 5

How to Break a Fast Like a Women

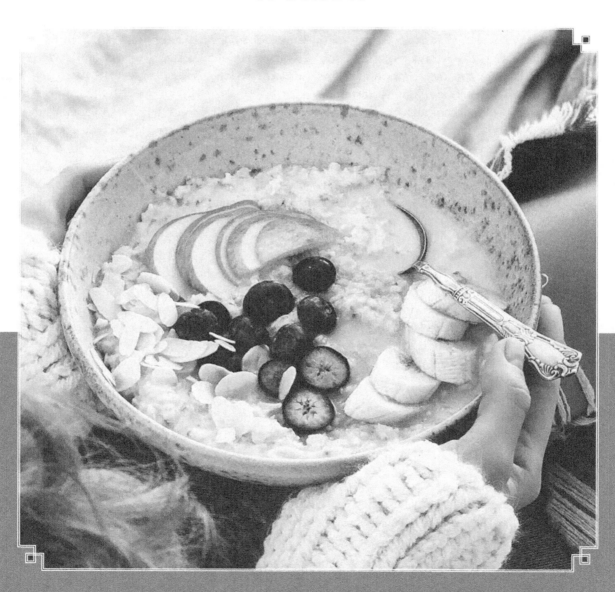

Till now, you have learned enough about fasting. You can confidently choose which fast is appropriate for you and what you should do while fasting in a 30-day cycle. However, there is a more complex yet easy subject we haven't touched yet. And the subject is how to break a fast like a woman. This might seem easier but it is truly not. Most people see fasting as an exercise, but as you deep dive into fasting you realize this is more of an art. Fasting was first used for healing and at that time breaking the fast was not a concern. The theory of breaking fast like a woman is that the results you get from fasting should stick around. And a huge part of it depends on what foods you intake for breaking the fast. There are 4 ways to break the fast. It depends on your goals and how you are going to break the fast. Just like you can choose the fasting length according to your goals, you can also determine the way of breaking your fast.

Microbiome Reset Foods

Fasting is the ultimate way to reset your microbiome. In a fasting state, your gut which has good bacteria can grow and help in the production of many hormones. So you have to break your fast with foods that are good for your gut bacteria. probiotics add more good bacteria to your gut and help overcome years of antibiotics and birth control pill effects.

Another type of food good for your microbiome is prebiotics. Prebiotics feed your microbes so they can grow and help you boost your hormone production. They can break down estrogen and it provides mood-enhancing neurotransmitters.

Polyphenol foods are an excellent choice for repairing the mucosal line in your guts. These foods will help you overcome low energy and chronic pain. Leaky gut and brain fog. You can combine all of these foods for the betterment of your microbiome health.

The below-mentioned foods are best for you if you want to reset your microbiome health

- Fermented yogurts, including coconut and dairy varieties
- Bone broth
- Sauerkraut
- Kombucha
- Seeds and seed oils
- Prebiotic-rich protein powders

Muscle Building Foods

Many people think that fasting breaks your muscles. This is a misconception that has been going around for years. What happens is that fasting your muscles releases stored sugar. This is very important for your muscles to release stored sugar and other toxins. Your muscles just shrink temporarily after fasting, what you can do is take protein to build your muscles stronger than before. It will keep you energized and help you stay strong. For meat eaters, choosing protein is very easy. Vegetarians also can break their fast with their favorite protein shake.

The below-mentioned foods are best for you if you want to build muscles

- Eggs
- Beef sticks
- Beef jerky
- Protein shakes such as pea, hemp, and whey concentrate
- Sliced deli meats (nitrite-free)
- Chicken breast
- Turkey
- Grass-fed beef
- High-protein vegetables such as peas, broccoli, sprouts, mushrooms, and brussels sprouts

- Chickpeas
- Lima beans
- Quinoa
- Avocado

- Avocado
- Raw nuts or nut butter
- Olives
- Bone broth

Fat Burning Foods

Out of all macronutrients in your body, fat stabilizes your blood sugar level the most. For that reason, it is a good idea to break a fast with fat if you are looking to burn the fat stored in your body. You can even take a small amount of fat in between your fast to burn fat more effectively. Taking a little amount of fat during your fast won't pull you out of fasting. But the hardest part about this is what kind of fat you have to eat. Foods that are primarily made of fat are called fat bombs. These fat bombs are ideal for taking. Making up new fat bombs can be difficult so go for pre-made fat bombs. Many companies provide the perfect fat bombs. This fat will provide you with energy to go through the day and kill your hunger at the same time.

Foods to break your fast with that keep you burning fat:

Follow Your Heart

Some say that your heart is connected to your taste buds. So breaking your fast with the food you love is a good idea. But what if you love foods that will destroy progress? Well, that is not possible because it will not undo the healing effects. Instead, you will feel the satisfaction of your favorite food. However, this has its own pros and cons. The advantage of following your heart is you will feel an instant satisfaction that will motivate you to fast. On the other hand, once you start eating your favorite food, all the healing effects in your body will immediately stop. So breaking your fast using the other 3 types of food is always the best choice.

Eating junk food as your fast-breaking food won't undo the healing but it is surely going to delay your goals. So breaking your fast using the other 3 types of food is always the best choice.

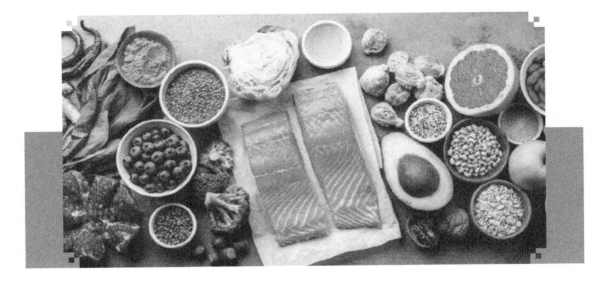

Chapter 6

How to Make Fasting Effortless

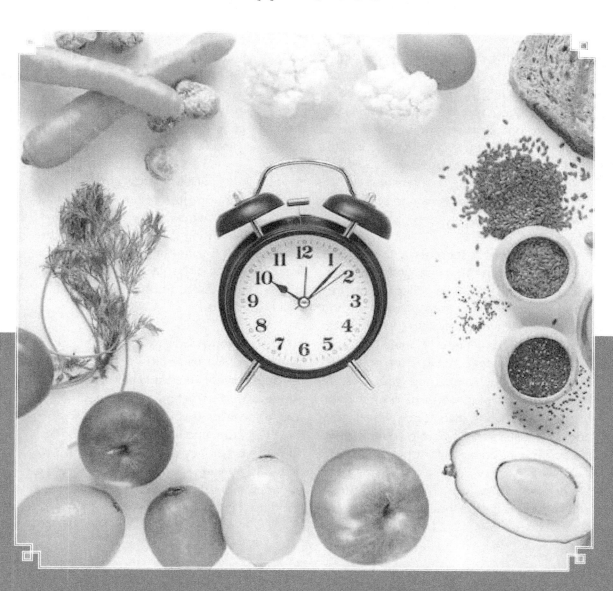

Fasting is a wonderful practice to make your body healthier and to live a healthy life. Till now, you have learned much about fasting. But now I am going to tell you how to make fasting effortless for you. Excited about how you are going to make these long fasts effortless?

Before that, you need to understand what I mean by effortless. The goal of healing is not always about speed, this is about the healing process is not all about speed. Healing takes time and if you have a chronic condition, it will take time to solve it. You have to be patient about it and live your life with fasting. The more you sync fasting with your life, the more opportunity you give your body to heal. And you have to practice, to master fasting. It is just like playing a new instrument, you can't just choose an instrument and start playing it. You have to learn how to play an instrument and after a lot of practice, you get good at it. Just like playing an instrument, fasting is also an art. It requires a lot of hard work and practice to master fasting.

If you are new at fasting, try a 17-hour fast and if you feel it is too much, go for 13 hours. The fact is no fast has failed. Each fast releases different hormones in your body and they target different goals. So do not be sad if you can not complete 17 hours but learn more about fasting. A big part of fasting depends on how motivated you are, the knowledge you gain works as a motivation as well. Here I will also teach you 9 easy hacks for fasting that will help you to fasting life easier and more comfortable,

So let's learn how you can make your fasts effortless and get a healthy body at the same time.

Handling Hunger

Hunger is the biggest problem for fasters. Everyone has to learn how to handle their hunger faster. To handle hunger, the first question you need to ask yourself is if you are truly hungry or just bored. Food is a mental state changer so many people subconsciously take food as a mood changer. To find out if you are hungry or bored, do things that make you happy. For example, play a song, dance, watch a movie, or call your favorite friends. Taking a nap can also be helpful in this situation. See if your hunger goes away or if you are still hungry, if you find yourself hungry try taking minerals. Hunger can also be caused by mineral imbalance so taking a boost of sodium, potassium, and magnesium is not a bad idea. Make sure they are unsweetened otherwise, they will spike your blood sugar.

If you find yourself hungry after taking minerals you can go for some fast snacks. Remember fat bombs? They can be perfect snacks while fasting to give your body a little energy and kill your hunger. Aside from fat bombs, you can also try taking some MCT oil in your tea or coffee to provide some fat to your body.

Another effective way to kill your hunger is by feeding your microbes in a fasted state. Because it is not your body cells that always demand food, sometimes your gut is the one asking for food. If you feed those microbes they will stop ending hunger signals. You can take prebiotics to kill your hunger. Take prebiotic powder with water, tea, or coffee, and remember that prebiotics only feed the good bacteria.

When To Use Coffee And Tea while Fasting

Drinking tea or coffee during fasting can be very beneficial unless you have a blood sugar problem. Ingredients available in coffee can stimulate autophagy which will do an extra favor during fasting. Try to buy organic coffee unless some coffees are full of pesticides that can spike your sugar level. If you find it hard to buy organic coffee, many companies sell organic coffee. Organic coffee is a popular concept now so it won't be hard for you to find organic coffee. The chemicals in other poor-quality coffees can keep you insulin-resistant and harm your fasting results.

Fasting-Friendly Tea Choices

Varieties of herbal teas are a great choice for those seeking a delicious, healthy, and calorie-free beverage. Different types of herbs in these teas can either boost metabolism or provide a calming effect on the nerves while also contributing positively to your physique.

GREEN TEA

Green tea is believed by researchers to trigger a thermogenic response in the body due to its plant compounds. This response leads to the conversion of fat molecules into energy, which are then eliminated from the body. Additionally, green tea aids in digestion thanks to its bitter components. To experience the slimming effects, you need to consume four cups of 150 ml each daily.

MATCHA TEA

Matcha tea, a specific type of green tea loaded with antioxidants and known for its anti-inflammatory properties, enhances fat burning through its catechin content. To prepare this beneficial blend, mix 1/2 teaspoon of matcha with 80 ml of hot water using a bamboo whisk.

TEFF TEA

Teff tea, a blend of various herbs and teas enriched with teff flour or teff seeds, is not easily found. Teff, a type of millet rich in fiber, can contribute to weight loss by keeping you feeling full.

ST. JOHN'S WORT TEA

St. John's Wort, known for its yellow flowers, is both a mood enhancer and a soul comforter, aiding in maintaining motivation during a diet. Moreover, it helps curb cravings. Prepare by steeping six teaspoons of St. John's Wort with two cinnamon sticks and two-star aniseed for 5-7 minutes.

WHITE TEA:

White tea is an excellent choice to support your body's defenses, which can weaken during dieting. It also promotes fat metabolism and has skin-firming flavonoids. It's most enjoyable in the afternoon. To make it, scald 3-4 heaped teaspoons of white tea leaves, and add fresh mint if desired, then steep for 2-5 minutes.

GINGER TEA

Ginger tea is rich in essential vitamins and minerals and can raise your body's operating temperature, thereby increasing metabolism. It also accelerates the production of stomach acid, aiding in faster digestion.

MATE TEA

Originating from South America, Mate tea, with effects similar to caffeine, revs up metabolism and reduces hunger. Steep Mate tea leaves for 7 minutes to prepare.

OOLONG TEA

Saponins in oolong tea support the breakdown of fats by the body's enzymes, allowing them to be eliminated without digestion. Caffeine in the tea also contributes to a boosted metabolism. This tea contains antioxidants that help detoxify the body and promote a healthy appearance.

ROOIBOS TEA

Tea from South Africa, rich in aromatic oils, can help suppress appetite, particularly the craving for sweets. For added flavor, consider combining it with a vanilla or cinnamon stick. Steep 2-3 teaspoons of rooibos for 5 minutes to experience these benefits.

Top 8 Fasting Hacks

1. Drink enough water

Fasting is not all about being motivated and not eating for hours. This is an art for what you need enough instruments for. Water is one of the most important elements that keeps you hydrated and helps you. Start your morning with a full 8-ounce glass of water. It will keep you hydrated and set a target for your body to drink more water throughout the day

2. Stay involved

Staying busy or staying involved in something is helpful in many situations. Fasting is no different, it will keep your mind away from fasting and help your body to increase hormone production.

3. Drink coffee or green tea

Drinking coffee can help to reduce the hunger signals from your body. It is a mild hunger suppressant. There is also evidence of green tea, black tea, and bone broth being good hunger suppressants and they will help you to control your appetite.

4. Ride with the hunger waves

As you have already noticed you are not hungry all the time. You are just hungry in waves, for some minutes. So whenever the hunger waves hit you drink a glass of water or a cup of hot coffee. You might even forget that you were hungry.

5. Keep it a secret

Sometimes it is a good idea to stay silent. And the same rule goes for fasting. When you tell people that are fasting many people will discourage you by saying harmful things about fasting. But the fact is they do not understand fasting as you do. So keep it a secret and surprise everyone with the fasting results

6. Take time

Fasting is a hard thing at first but it gets easier with time. So take time and at least take 1 month. If you can continue the fasting cycle for a month, you will see the dramatic changes and understand the beauty of fasting. Otherwise, you will get discouraged and might stop fasting forever.

7. Follow a nutritious diet when not fasting

You obviously can not eat much on the days you are fasting. But do not jump into a junk food festival in your non-fasting days. Follow a nutritious diet so you can give enough nutrients to your organs.

8. Make fasting part of your life

This is the most important hack I can offer. For permanent results and to live a healthy life you have to stick to fasting. You do not have to change your life for fasting, instead set a fasting schedule that fits your daily activities. There will be times when it will become impossible for you to fast like festivals, wedding holidays and many more. So eat on the special days and cover them by fasting on the days you do not have to eat much.

Chapter 7

Handling Detox Symptoms

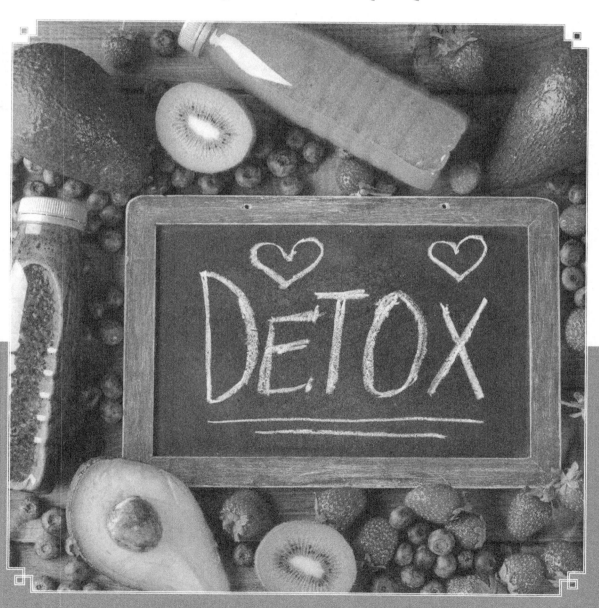

Fasting is a good way to detox harmful compounds stored in your body. But sometimes, some detox symptoms can make you suffer for a short time. One of the examples is keto flu, which occurs when you get ketosis for the first time. Some symptoms of keto flu are rashes, muscle aches, fever, constipation, fatigue, brain fog and many more. These symptoms can be disturbing but you have to face it calmly. Because ketosis will have a healing effect on your body which will slowly remove these symptoms. Symptoms during fasting prove that ketosis is working on your body. These symptoms occur because your body is increasing its heat to kill those bacteria. Also, rashes can appear as your body is pushing those germs away through your skin. In simple words, these symptoms are a sign of ketosis healing your body.

If you are facing strong detox symptoms you follow three things. The first thing you need to do is bring variation in your fasting. Remember the 30-day fasting cycle? Detox symptoms do not appear when you frequently vary your fast. You can skip one or two days to give your body the chance to surge in those toxins.

The second method is to open up your detox pathways so the toxins can move easily. These pathways include the gut, kidney, liver, lymph, and skin. As 17-hour or longer fasts can cause you to have detox symptoms, follow these below-mentioned hacks to open up your detox pathways.

Sweating

Sweating can move the circulation and open up the pores of your body. It will help push the toxins out of your body. A good amount of sweating daily can dramatically help you

detox

Dry Brushing

Dry brushing your hair with a hard brush can exfoliate your skin and open pores for the toxin to exit the body.

Lymph Massage

Your lymph carries away the toxins from your organs. A good lymphatic massage is very helpful in getting your lymph moving again. You can also jump up and down for your lymphatic system to move.

Epsom salt bath

If you are looking for rashes, headaches, and joint pain to go away try this method. Magnesium mixed with warm water works magically to get rid of these symptoms. When autophagy starts, it pushes toxins out of the pathways, and to grab those toxins you use a binder. Binders like zeolite or activated charcoal are good for detoxing.

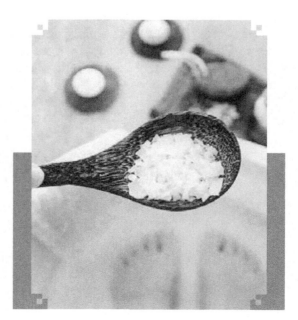

Chapter 8

What Breaks Your Fast?

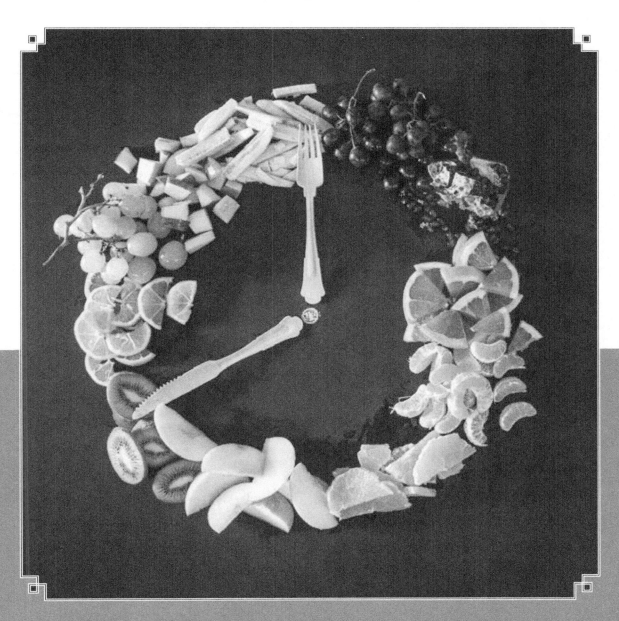

When you are fasting you need at least anything to keep you going. You can not eat or drink everything while fasting or your body will step aside from the fasting state. Many drinks do not break you fast but it entirely depends on your body. Because if your blood sugar rises and switches to the sugar-burner system, it is when your fast breaks. So what you need to do is keep your sugar level low and stay in a fast state. Remember that it takes you to starve 8 hours before reaching the fasting state. Anything that raises your sugar level breaks your fast. Although some drinks do not increase your blood sugar and keep you in a fasted state.

However, what might pull you out of a fasted state might help me go through the day. This happens because everyone's body needs are different and you will need to test these drinks using a blood sugar test.

- Alcohol
- Sweeteners in your coffee or tea
- Diet drinks
- Gatorade
- Coffee creamers
- Sodas

Along with foods that pull you out of a fasting state, some foods keep you in a fasting state. Here is a list of foods that keep you in a fasted state and provide you with energy to keep going through the day.

- Medications
- Supplements
- Coffee with full-fat milk
- Black coffee
- Oils, including flaxseed and MCT
- Tea
- Mineral water

Blood Sugar Test

There is a very easy way to test which drinks pull you out of the fasted state. The first step is to take a blood sugar reader and do a glucose check. Now remember the reading and drink the drink you want to taste. After you have drunk it, wait for 30 minutes and take a glucose reading again. If your blood sugar level is the same or the first reading is lower than the last reading you are still in the fasted state. Vice versa, if the second reading is higher than the first time, know that the drink has pulled you out of a fasting state and you are now in a sugar burner state.

Some foods or food ingredients pull you out of a fasted state. And here is a list of foods that pull you out of a fasting state.

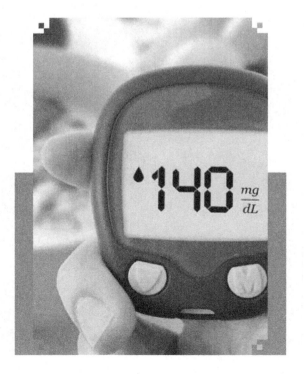

Chapter 9

Recipes

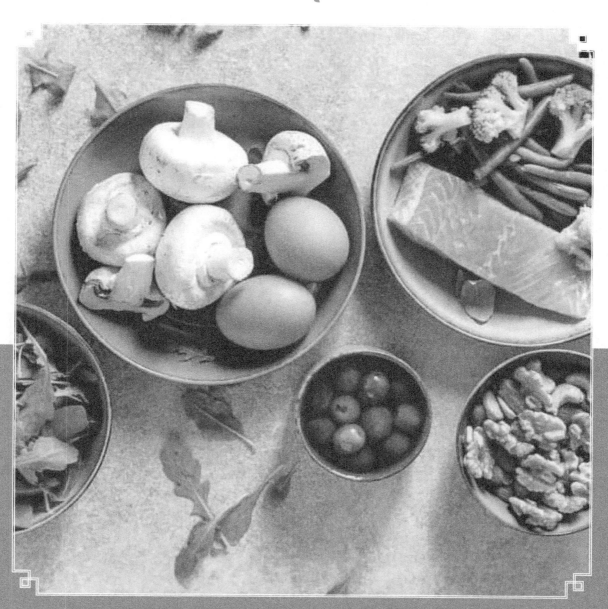

Your diet during this 30-day fast plan is very important. The foods you intake should be synched with your body's nutrient demands. But that does not mean you have to eat boring boiled food all the time. Instead pairing with tasty food will help you fast and gain your goals effortlessly. Below are some amazing nutrient and yummy recipes to excite both your taste buds and hormones. But one thing you need to know is these recipes are not the only thing you can eat. Be more creative and do not be shy to try other foods. Many people naturally shy away from the food they do not like. But remember that diversity of food choices only helps you live a healthier life.

Ketobiotic Recipes

Cream Cheese Pancakes

Prep time: 5 minutes | Cook time: 12 minutes | Makes 4 (6-inch) pancakes

Cream Cheese Pancakes can be a suitable choice for an intermittent fasting eating plan for several reasons. These pancakes are low in carbohydrates, as they do not contain traditional flour, making them compatible with fasting periods. The combination of cream cheese, eggs, and erythritol provides a decent amount of protein and healthy fats, which can help you stay full and satisfied during your eating window. Furthermore, the absence of refined sugars ensures these pancakes won't lead to spikes in blood sugar, which is important for intermittent fasters seeking stable energy levels.

- 2 ounces cream cheese (¼ cup), softened
- 2 large eggs
- 1 teaspoon granulated erythritol
- ½ teaspoon ground cinnamon
- 1 tablespoon butter, for the pan

1. Place the cream cheese, eggs, sweetener, and cinnamon in a small blender and blend for 30 seconds, or until smooth. Let the batter rest for 2 minutes.

2. Heat the butter in a 10-inch nonstick skillet over medium heat until bubbling. Pour ¼ cup of the batter into the pan and tilt the pan in a circular motion to create a thin pancake about 6 inches in diameter. Cook for 2 minutes, or until the center is no longer glossy. Flip and cook for 1 minute on the other side. Remove and repeat with the rest of the batter, making a total of 4 pancakes.

PER SERVING

Calories: 395 | Fat: 35g | Protein: 17g | Carbs: 3g | Fiber: 0g

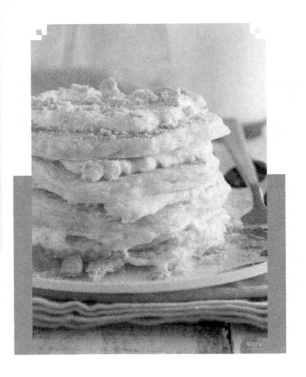

Open-Faced Tacos

Prep time: 10 minutes | Cook time:20 minutes
|Serves 4

This recipe is a good choice for intermittent fasting because it offers a balance of protein and healthy fats while minimizing carbohydrates. The use of chicken thighs and ground beef provides a substantial protein source, which can help promote feelings of fullness during the fasting window. The healthy fats from avocado or coconut oil can also support satiety.The absence of traditional tortillas reduces carb intake, which can be beneficial for those following intermittent fasting, especially during the fasting hours. The combination of protein, fats, and minimal carbs in this recipe can help stabilize blood sugar levels, preventing energy crashes.

Tortillas:

- 2 pounds boneless, skinless chicken thighs
- ⅓ cup avocado oil, or ⅓ cup coconut oil

Filling:

- 1 pound ground beef
- 1 clove garlic, minced
- 1½ teaspoons chili powder
- ½ teaspoon ground cumin
- ½ teaspoon paprika
- ½ teaspoon finely ground sea salt
- ¼ teaspoon red pepper flakes
- ⅛ teaspoon ground black pepper

Toppings:

- ⅔ cup shredded cheddar cheese (dairy-free or regular)
- 1 small tomato, diced
- 4 leaves green leaf lettuce, chopped

1. Place the chicken thighs on a sheet of parchment paper. Using a meat mallet, pound the thighs until they're ¼ inch (6 mm) thick.
2. Heat the oil in a large frying pan over medium-high heat. Add the chicken and cook for 10 minutes, then flip and cook for another 10 minutes, or until each side is golden and the internal temperature reaches 165°F.
3. Meanwhile, place the ground beef, garlic, chili powder, cumin, paprika, salt, red pepper flakes, and black pepper in another large frying pan. Cook over medium heat until the meat is no longer pink, about 10 minutes, stirring to crumble it as it cooks.
4. To assemble, place the cooked chicken "tortillas" on serving plates and top with the ground beef filling, then the shredded cheese, diced tomato, and chopped lettuce. Dig in!

PER SERVING

Calories: 832 | Total Fat: 60 g | Carbs: 5 g | Fiber: 4 g |Protein: 68 g

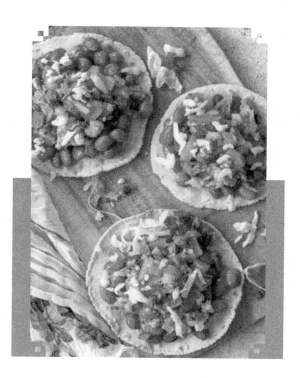

Full Meal Deal

Prep time: 10 minutes | Cook time:3 minutes |Serves 4

The "Full Meal Deal" recipe aligns well with an intermittent fasting eating plan due to its balanced nutrient profile, offering healthy fats from avocado and avocado oil, leafy greens from fresh spinach, and flavorful chimichurri sauce. This combination ensures a well-rounded mix of nutrients, promoting satiety and stable energy levels during the fasting period while being low in refined carbohydrates. With quick preparation, it's convenient for intermittent fasters, and the addition of chimichurri sauce makes it a flavorful and enjoyable meal for the eating window. This recipe can be a beneficial choice for those following intermittent fasting, providing a nutritious and satisfying meal that supports the fasting regimen.

- 2 Mug Biscuits
- 1 large avocado, peeled, pitted, and mashed (about 6 oz/170 g of flesh)
- 1 tablespoon avocado oil
- 2 cups (140 g) fresh spinach
- ½ cup (105 g) Chimichurri

1. Cut the biscuits in half and set each half on a separate plate. Top each half with an equal portion of the mashed avocado.
2. Place the oil in a medium-sized frying pan over medium heat. Add the spinach and sauté until lightly wilted, about 3 minutes.
3. Place the wilted spinach on top of the avocado, then drizzle each serving with 2 tablespoons of chimichurri. Enjoy immediately.

PER SERVING

Calories: 358 | Fat: 33.8 g| Carbs: 6.5 g | Fiber: 3.3 g |Protein: 7.1 g

Bacon-Wrapped Avocado Fries

Prep time: 10 minutes | Cook time:18 minutes |Serves 4

Bacon-Wrapped Avocado Fries, a tasty choice for an intermittent fasting eating plan, offer a satisfying option rich in healthy fats from avocados and bacon, promoting satiety and helping maintain steady energy levels during fasting periods. Low in carbohydrates and quick to prepare, they align with the principles of intermittent fasting. The combination of crispy bacon and creamy avocado provides a flavorful and enjoyable experience, but it's important to exercise portion control due to its calorie density to avoid overeating. While it can be part of an intermittent fasting regimen, it's advisable to balance it with other nutrient-rich foods to ensure overall nutritional adequacy.

- 2 medium Hass avocados, peeled and pitted (about 8 oz/220 g of flesh)
- 16 strips bacon (about 1 lb/455 g), cut in half lengthwise

1. Cut each avocado into 8 fry-shaped pieces, making a total of 16 fries.
2. Wrap each avocado fry in 2 half-strips of bacon. Once complete, place in a large frying pan.
3. Set the pan over medium heat and cover with a splash guard. Fry for 6 minutes on each side and on the bottom, or until crispy, for a total of 18 minutes.
4. Remove from the heat and enjoy immediately!

PER SERVING

Calories: 723 | Fat: 58.3 g | Carbs: 6.4 g | Fiber: 3.7 g |Protein: 43.2 g

Cabbage & Sausage with Bacon

Prep time: 10 minutes | Cook time:25 minutes |Serves 4

Cabbage & Sausage with Bacon is a hearty recipe that can be beneficial for an intermittent fasting eating plan. This dish combines bacon, cabbage, onion, garlic, and chorizo, offering a balance of proteins, healthy fats, and vegetables that supports satiety and helps maintain energy levels during the eating window. With relatively low carbohydrates, it aligns with the goal of preventing blood sugar spikes and crashes. Additionally, its quick preparation time makes it convenient for intermittent fasters looking for a wholesome, filling meal without extensive cooking. The flavorful combination of bacon, chorizo, and cabbage enhances the eating experience.

- 6 strips bacon (about 6 oz/170 g), diced
- 1 small red onion, diced
- 4 cloves garlic, minced
- 1 small head green cabbage (about 1⅓ lbs/600 g), cored and thinly sliced
- 12 ounces (340 g) Mexican-style fresh (raw) chorizo, thinly sliced
- ¼ cup (60 ml) beef bone broth

1. Place the bacon, onion, and garlic in a large frying pan and sauté over medium heat until the bacon begins to crisp, about 10 minutes.
2. Add the cabbage, sausage slices, and broth. Cover and cook for 15 minutes, until the cabbage is fork-tender and the sausage is cooked through.
3. Remove the lid, divide among 4 dinner plates, and enjoy!

PER SERVING

Calories: 523 | Fat: 43.8 g| Carbs: 12 g | Fiber: 4 g | Protein: 20 g

Cheesy Broccoli

Prep time: 5 minutes | Cook time: 30 minutes | Serves 4

Cheesy Broccoli can be integrated into an intermittent fasting eating plan with certain considerations. This dish, featuring nutrient-rich broccoli, low carbohydrates, and healthy fats from grass-fed butter, ghee, or coconut oil, supports satiety and prevents blood sugar fluctuations. Its quick preparation is convenient for intermittent fasters, and the flavorful blend of cheddar and Parmesan cheese enhances the taste. However, portion control is essential due to the calorie and fat content from the cheese. While Cheesy Broccoli can be part of an intermittent fasting regimen, it should be enjoyed in moderation and balanced with other nutrient-rich foods to fit within your daily calorie intake.

- 1 pound broccoli florets (fresh or frozen)
- 4 tablespoonsgrass-fed butter,ghee, or coconut oil
- ½ teaspoon sea salt
- 1 cup shredded cheddar cheese
- ¼ cup freshly grated Parmesan cheese

1. Preheat the oven to 400°F.
2. Bring 1 inch of water to a boil in a large pot over medium-high heat. Add in the broccoli, cover, and cook for 5 minutes.
3. Drain the broccoli and put it in agreased medium casserole dish.
4. Add the butter and mix it together well. Top with the salt and cheese.
5. Bake for 20 minutes, or until the cheese begins to brown.

PER SERVING

Calories: 297 | Fat: 25.1g | Protein: 12.9g | Carbs: 8.2g | Fiber: 3g

Coconut Curry and Ginger Chicken Meatballs

Prep time: 5 minutes | Cook time: 30 minutes | Serves 4

Coconut Curry and Ginger Chicken Meatballs offer several advantages for an intermittent fasting eating plan. This dish is rich in protein from ground chicken, promoting satiety during the eating window. Additionally, its quick preparation time is convenient for intermittent fasters looking for a protein-packed meal without extended cooking. The flavorful combination of Thai curry paste, ginger, and garlic makes it a satisfying and enjoyable dish.

- 1 poundground chicken
- 1 inch fresh ginger, peeled and minced
- 2garlic cloves, minced
- ½ teaspoon sea salt
- 1 tablespoon coconut aminos
- 2 tablespoons coconut oil
- 1 (4-ounce) can red curry paste
- 1 (15-ounce) can full-fat coconut milk

1. In a medium bowl, mix theground chicken,ginger,garlic, salt, and coconut aminos. Scoop out tablespoonfuls of the meat mixture and roll into 1-inch balls. Repeat, using the rest of the meat.
2. Melt the coconut oil in a large skillet over medium heat and add the meatballs, leaving space in between. Remove them as they are cooked to a plate.
3. Add the curry paste to the skillet and toast for 1 minute. Pour in the coconut milk and mix together. Return the meatballs to the skillet and cook for 4 to 5 minutes. Serve warm.

PER SERVING

Calories: 571 | Fat: 44g | Protein: 35.1g | Carbs: 8.4g | Fiber: 0g

Salmon Salad Cups

Prep time: 10 minutes | Cook time:5 minutes |Serves 4

The Salmon Salad Cups recipe is a suitable choice for an intermittent fasting eating plan due to its combination of protein and healthy fats from salmon, which can promote a sense of fullness, while being low in carbohydrates due to the use of lettuce leaves as cups. This reduces the potential for blood sugar spikes, making it a good option for intermittent fasting. Its quick and easy preparation aligns well with time-restricted eating, and the inclusion of horseradish, dill, lemon juice, and seasonings adds flavorful variety. To ensure it adheres to your fasting schedule, consume it within your designated eating window and consider its place within your overall daily macronutrient balance.

- 12 ounces (340 g) canned salmon (no salt added)
- 3 tablespoons prepared horseradish
- 1 tablespoon chopped fresh dill
- 2 teaspoons lemon juice
- ½ teaspoon finely ground sea salt
- ½ teaspoon ground black pepper
- 12 butter lettuce leaves (from 1 head)
- ½ cup (105 g) mayonnaise

1. Place the salmon, horseradish, dill, lemon juice, salt, and pepper in a medium-sized bowl. Stir until the ingredients are fully incorporated.
2. Set the lettuce leaves on a serving plate. Fill each leaf with 2 tablespoons of the salmon salad mixture and top with 2 teaspoons of mayonnaise.

PER SERVING

Calories: 314 |Total Fat: 26.5 g | Carbs: 4.4 g | Fiber: 1.1 g | Protein: 14.6 g

Pepper Sausage Fry

Prep time: 5 minutes | Cook time:20 minutes |Serves 4

The Pepper Sausage Fry recipe is suitable for an intermittent fasting eating plan due to its balance of protein and healthy fats from smoked sausages and avocado or coconut oil, promoting satiety within the eating window, while also being low in carbohydrates. This lower carb content can assist in maintaining steady blood sugar levels, which aligns with intermittent fasting. Its quick preparation and cooking time make and parsley adds taste variety. To ensure it fits your intermittent fasting schedule, enjoy it within your designated eating hours, and consider its place in your overall daily macronutrient balance.

- ¼ cup (60 ml) avocado oil, or ¼ cup (55 g) coconut oil
- 12 ounces (340 g) smoked sausages, thinly sliced
- 1 small green bell pepper, thinly sliced
- 1 small red bell pepper, thinly sliced
- 1½ teaspoons garlic powder
- 1 teaspoon dried oregano leaves
- 1 teaspoon paprika
- ¼ teaspoon finely ground sea salt
- ¼ teaspoon ground black pepper
- ¼ cup (17 g) chopped fresh parsley

1. Heat the oil in a large frying pan over medium-low heat until it shimmers.
2. When the oil is shimmering, add the rest of the ingredients, except the parsley. Cover and cook for 15 minutes, until the bell peppers are fork-tender.
3. Remove the lid and continue to cook for 5 to 6 minutes, until the liquid evaporates.
4. Remove from the heat, stir in the parsley, and serve.

PER SERVING

Calories: 411 | Total Fat: 38.3 g | Carbs: 6.3 g | Fiber: 1.5 g | Protein: 11.1 g

Keto Chocolate Frosty

Prep time: 5 minutes | Cook time: 35 minutes | Serves 1

The Keto Chocolate Frosty can be a suitable option for an intermittent fasting eating plan, provided that it's consumed in moderation due to its calorie content. This dessert is low in carbohydrates, making it beneficial for avoiding blood sugar fluctuations during fasting. It includes healthy fats from full-fat coconut milk and almond butter, which support satiety and help maintain energy levels during the eating window. With a quick and straightforward preparation, it's a convenient choice for intermittent fasters seeking a dessert without prolonged cooking. Additionally, its use of stevia as a sweetener adheres to a keto diet, ensuring low carbohydrate and sugar content.

- 1 cup full fat coconut milk
- 2 tablespoons cocoa powder
- 1 tablespoon almond butter
- 1 teaspoon vanilla extract
- 1 tablespoon stevia (about 5 packets)

1. In a medium bowl, whisk together all the with an electric hand mixer, stand mixer, or a hand-whisk for 30 seconds, or until the are fully incorporated, thick, and creamy.
2. Freeze for 30 minutes. Whisk again for smoothness and enjoy.

PER SERVING

Calories: 579 | Fat: 58.6g | Protein: 9.9g | Carbs: 15.8g | Fiber: 4.8g

Hormone Feasting Recipes

Sweet Potato Pancakes

Prep time: 10 minutes | Cook time: 25 minutes | Serves 4

Sweet Potato Pancakes, with their complex carbohydrates from sweet potatoes, protein from eggs and Greek yogurt, and minimal added sugar from maple syrup, can be a suitable choice for an intermittent fasting eating plan. These pancakes feature whole ingredients, promoting the consumption of unprocessed and nutritious foods during the eating window.

- 1 sweet potato
- 1 tsp olive oil
- 1 egg
- 4 egg whites
- 1 cup fat-free greek yogurt
- 1/2 cup oats
- 1 tsp maple syrup
- 1 banana, sliced

1. Rinse sweet potato and add to a microwaveable sandwich bag with olive oil.
2. Microwave for 12 minutes.
3. Remove and allow to cool before removing the skin from the sweet potato with a sharp knife.
4. If you don't have a microwave, simply pierce sweet potato with a fork and add to a hot oven for 20-30 minutes or until soft.
5. Put the oats into a blender and blend to a fine powder, then place into a bowl.
6. Place the sweet potato in the blender and blend until smooth, and then mix with the powdered oats.
7. Pour roughly a quarter of the batter into the pan and cook for 1-2 minutes.
8. Enjoy hot with sliced banana to serve (optional).
9. Use the same method for the rest of your batter.

PER SERVING

Calories: 376 | Protein: 16g | Carbs: 45g | Fat: 15g

Easy Beef Stew

Prep time: 10 minutes | Cook time: 25 minutes | Serves 4

Bodybuilding Beef Stew, rich in protein from lean beef and complex carbohydrates from sweet potatoes, is a compatible choice for an intermittent fasting eating plan. The inclusion of herbs and spices enhances both flavor and potential health benefits, while avoiding refined carbohydrates helps maintain stable blood sugar levels.

- 1 tbsp of extra virgin olive oil
- 8 oz lean beef, cubed
- 1 onion, diced
- 4 cups of water
- 1 tsp cumin
- 1 tsp turmeric
- 2 sweet potatoes, peeled and cubed
- 1 red bell pepper, roughly chopped
- 1 bay leaf

1. Heat the olive oil in a skillet over a medium to high heat.
2. Add the beef and cook for 5 minutes or until browned on each side.
3. Add the vegetables and garlic to the slow cooker and pour in the water.
4. Now add the herbs, spices and bay leaf.
5. Then cover the slow cooker and cook for at least 8 hours or overnight.
6. Plate up and serve when ready to eat!

PER SERVING

Calories: 372 | Protein: 25g | Carbs: 42g | Fat: 12g

Cherry Protein Porridge

Prep time: 10 minutes | Cook time: 25 minutes | Serves 4

Cherry Protein Porridge, featuring rolled oats, cherries, vanilla protein powder, and almond milk, can align with an intermittent fasting eating plan while catering to the protein needs of bodybuilders. The combination of oats and protein powder offers a blend of carbohydrates and protein, which can aid in post-workout recovery during the eating window.

- 2 cups rolled oats
- 1/2 cup cherries
- 2 scoops vanilla protein powder
- 4 cups almond milk

1. Mix the oats with the almond milk in a large bowl.
2. Add to a pan on the stove over a medium heat until it starts to bubble slightly but not boil.
3. Alternatively place in the microwave for 1.5 minutes.
4. Remove from the pan and return to the large bowl.
5. Stir in the protein powder until there are no lumps left.
6. Top with cherries and serve.

PER SERVING

Calories: 370 | Protein: 27g | Carbs: 41g | Fat: 11g

Chili Beef & Mango Salsa

Prep time: 10 minutes | Cook time: 25 minutes | Serves 4

Chili Beef & Mango Salsa, a balanced meal with lean ground beef and a fresh mango salsa, can be a suitable choice for those following an intermittent fasting eating plan, provided that portion control is observed to meet specific calorie goals. The combination of lean protein from beef and complex carbohydrates from quinoa contributes to satiety and sustained energy during the eating window. The use of fresh ingredients such as cherry tomatoes, mango, and cilantro aligns with the goal of consuming nutrient-rich foods within the eating window.

- 1 red onion, diced
- 1/2 red bell pepper, diced
- 1 garlic clove, minced
- 10 oz lean ground beef
- 1 red chili, finely diced
- 1/4 cup kidney beans
- 2 tbsp extra virgin olive oil
- 1/2 cup cherry tomatoes, diced
- 1/4 cup mango, diced
- 1/2 lime, juiced
- 1 cup quinoa
- 1 tbsp fresh cilantro

1. Bring a pan of water to the boil and add quinoa for 20 minutes.
2. Meanwhile, add 1 tbsp oil to a pan and heat on a medium to high heat.
3. Add the half the onions, pepper, chili and garlic and sauté for 5 minutes until soft.
4. Add the beef to the pan and stir until browned.
5. Now add the kidney beans and the water, cover and turn the heat down a little to simmer for 20 minutes.
6. Meanwhile, drain the water from the quinoa, add the lid and steam while the chili is cooking.
7. Prepare the salsa by mixing the rest of the onion, tomatoes, lime juice, cilantro and mango.
8. Serve chili hot with the quinoa and salsa.

PER SERVING

Calories: 591 | Protein: 39g | Carbs: 51g | Fat: 27g

Spicy Mexican Bean Stew

Prep time: 10 minutes | Cook time: 25 minutes | Serves 4

Spicy Mexican Bean Stew, featuring chickpeas, cannellini beans, chorizo, and a spicy kick, can be considered for an intermittent fasting eating plan, with caution regarding portion sizes and calorie intake. The inclusion of beans provides fiber and protein, promoting satiety during the eating window. While the stew contains chorizo and olive oil, it's essential to control portions and balance the meal with nutrient-rich foods to fit within specific calorie goals during intermittent fasting. The addition of red chilis and paprika enhances the flavor and aligns with the aim of incorporating spices to make dishes more interesting within the eating window.

- 8oz canned chick peas, drained
- 8oz canned cannellini beans, drained
- 8oz of tinned chopped tomatoes
- 2 tbsp olive oil
- 1 chopped red onion
- 6oz of sliced chorizo
- 3 red chopped chillis
- 1 tbsp paprika

1. Heat a large pan on a medium heat with 1 tbsp olive oil, and cook the onion and chorizo for 5 minutes until lightly golden.
2. Tip in the chickpeas with the cannellini beans and stir until heated through.
3. Add the tin of chopped tomatoes and paprika and cover to let simmer for 5-10 minutes.
4. Serve – recommended with crusty brown bread, couscous or brown rice for a winter warmer!

PER SERVING

Calories: 395 | Protein: 20g | Carbs: 45g | Fat: 15g

Zucchini Pasta Salad

Prep time: 5 minutes | Cook time:5 minutes |Serves 4

The Zucchini Pasta Salad recipe can be a suitable choice for an intermittent fasting eating plan. It offers low carbohydrates by replacing traditional pasta with zucchini, aiding in stable blood sugar levels. Zucchini provides fiber and essential nutrients while being low in calories, contributing to satiety during the eating window. The addition of pine nuts and olives adds healthy fats and some protein, further promoting a sense of fullness. With quick preparation, it's time-efficient for those adhering to time-restricted eating. The choice of creamy Italian dressing or other creamy salad dressings can be customized, but it's important to consider the dressing's calorie content and overall macronutrient balance to ensure it aligns with your fasting schedule. Enjoy it within your designated eating hours.

- 4 medium zucchinis, spiral sliced
- 12 ounces pitted black olives, cut in half lengthwise
- 1 pint cherry tomatoes, cut in half lengthwise
- ½ cup pine nuts
- ¼ cup plus 2 tablespoons sesame seeds
- ⅔ cup creamy Italian dressing or other creamy salad dressing of choice

1. Place all the ingredients in a large mixing bowl.
2. Toss to coat, then divide evenly between 4 serving plates or bowls.

PER SERVING

Calories: 562 | Total Fat: 53 g | Saturated Fat: 6.3 g | Carbs: 22 g | Fiber: 8.5 g |Protein: 8.9 g

Smoked Trout Fish Cakes

Prep time: 10 minutes | Cook time: 25 minutes | Serves 4

Smoked Trout Fish Cakes, with their combination of sweet potatoes, leeks, dill, and smoked trout, can be considered for an intermittent fasting eating plan, emphasizing the importance of portion control and mindful calorie consumption. The inclusion of sweet potatoes introduces complex carbohydrates, contributing to sustained energy during the eating window. While the dish contains smoked trout and olive oil, it's vital to monitor portions and balance the meal with nutrient-rich foods to fit within specific calorie goals during intermittent fasting.

- 2 large sweet potatoes, peeled and cubed
- 3 tbsp extra virgin olive oil
- 1 leek, chopped
- 4 tsp dill, chopped
- 1 tbsp grated orange peel
- 1 pack smoked trout, sliced
- 1/3 cup low fat greek yogurt (optional)

1. Preheat oven to 325°f/150°c/Gas Mark 3.
2. Lightly grease 2 ramekins or circular baking dishes with a little olive oil.
3. Heat the rest of the oil in a skillet over medium heat, and sauté the leeks and the potatoes for 5 minutes.
4. Lower the heat and cook for another 10 minutes until tender.
5. Add the dill, orange peel and the trout and mix well.
6. Fill the ramekins with half the mixture each, patting to compact.
7. Bake for 15 minutes and remove.

PER SERVING

Calories: 529 | Protein: 23g | Carbs: 47g | Fat: 26g

Bulgur Wheat, Feta Cheese & Quinoa Salad

Prep time: 10 minutes | Cook time: 25 minutes | Serves 4

Bulgur Wheat, Feta Cheese & Quinoa Salad, featuring a blend of bulgur wheat, quinoa, chickpeas, feta cheese, and fresh ingredients, can align with an intermittent fasting eating plan, with an emphasis on portion control and calorie awareness. The dish offers a combination of whole grains, protein, and healthy fats, contributing to satiety and a nutrient-rich eating experience. The use of pesto, lemon juice, and parsley enhances the salad's flavor and aligns with the aim of making meals enjoyable within the eating window.

- 1/2 cup of bulgur wheat, uncooked
- 1/2 cup of cooked quinoa
- 16oz of chickpeas, drained
- 2oz of feta cheese, crumbled
- 1 cup cherry tomatoes, chopped
- ½ jar of pesto
- 3 tbsp of fresh lemon juice
- 2 tbsp of fresh parsley, minced
- 1/4 tsp of black pepper
- 1 onion, sliced thinly
- 2 cups of water, boiling

1. Mix bulgur wheat with boiling water in a large-sized bowl. Cover and set aside for half an hour before draining.
2. Add lemon juice and pesto. Stir using a whisk.
3. Combine pesto mixture, bulgur, quinoa, feta, tomatoes, green onions, chickpeas, pepper, parsley in a large bowl. Gently toss to mix well.
4. Serve.

PER SERVING

Calories: 350 | Protein: 15g | Carbs: 50g | Fat: 15g

Shrimp Curry

Prep time: 15 minutes | Cook time:30 minutes |Serves 4

The Shrimp Curry recipe can be a suitable option for an intermittent fasting eating plan. It provides protein from shrimp and healthy fats from coconut oil or ghee, promoting a sense of fullness within the eating window. While it incorporates riced cauliflower as a lower-carb alternative to rice, it's important to be mindful of the overall carbohydrate content, including that from the curry paste. The inclusion of nutrient-rich ingredients like fennel, ginger, and cilantro enhances the meal's flavors and nutritional value, making it more satisfying. With a relatively quick preparation and cook time for a curry, it aligns well with time-restricted eating. To ensure it aligns with your fasting schedule, consume it within your designated eating hours and monitor the carb content, adjusting portion sizes if needed.

- ⅓ cup coconut oil or ghee, or ⅓ cup (80 ml) avocado oil
- 1 small white onion, sliced
- 1 small fennel bulb, sliced
- 3 tablespoons red curry paste
- 1 piece fresh ginger root, minced
- ¾ teaspoon finely ground sea salt
- 1 can lite coconut milk
- 1 pound medium shrimp, peeled, deveined, and tails removed
- 2 cups riced cauliflower
- ½ cup fresh cilantro leaves and stems, for serving

1. Heat the oil in a large saucepan over medium heat. Add the onion, fennel, curry paste, ginger, and salt. Sauté for 10 minutes, or until fragrant.
2. Transfer the sautéed onion mixture to a blender or food processor. Add the coconut milk and blend until smooth.
3. Return the mixture to the saucepan and add the shrimp and riced cauliflower. Cover and bring to a light boil over medium-high heat. Once lightly boiling, reduce the heat to medium-low and simmer for 20 minutes, until the cauliflower is soft.
4. Divide the curry among 4 bowls. Top with the cilantro and serve.

PER SERVING

Calories: 499 | Total Fat: 37.1 g | Saturated Fat: 29.8 g |Carbs: 14.2 g | Fiber: 3.4 g | Protein: 27.2 g

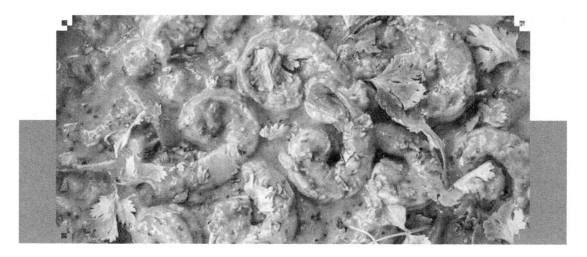

Steak & Sweet Potato Fries

Prep time: 10 minutes | Cook time: 25 minutes | Serves 4

Muscle Building Steak & Sweet Potato Fries, with its combination of sirloin steak, sweet potato fries, and salad, can be a fitting choice for individuals pursuing muscle-building goals within an intermittent fasting eating plan. The inclusion of steak provides high-quality protein, supporting muscle development and satiety during the eating window. Sweet potatoes offer complex carbohydrates for sustained energy. The use of olive oil, balsamic vinegar, and black pepper adds flavor to the dish and aligns with the goal of enhancing the taste of meals during the eating window.

- 4oz of sirloin steak
- 8oz of sweet potatoes cut into chips
- 1 tbsp olive oil
- 1 chopped red onion
- 1 bag of pre-washed salad
- 1 tbsp of balsamic vinegar
- a pinch of black pepper

1. Pre-Heat oven (375°F/190 °C/Gas Mark 5).
2. Get a baking tray, spread the chips out and bake for around 25 minutes.
3. While the chips are cooking, get a large frying pan and heat the olive oil on a medium heat.
4. Pepper the steaks and add to the pan. Fry the steaks for 6 minutes in total, turning the steaks once halfway through.
5. Take the steak and leave to cool.
6. Get a large bowl and add the salad and chopped onion. Drizzle with the vinegar and serve with the potatoes and steak.
7. the cheese and pine nuts and let the cheese melt for a further 4–5 minutes.
8. Plate up and serve.

PER SERVING

Calories: 418 | Protein: 29g | Carbs: 39g | Fat: 15g

Break Your Fast Recipes

Rhubarb Bombs

Prep time: 2 hours |Cook time: 0 minutes |Serves 10

Rhubarb Bombs, with a mix of ghee, coconut cream, almond butter and stevia, can potentially align with an intermittent fasting eating plan when consumed mindfully. These treats offer a blend of fats and minimal added sugars, which can be suitable for individuals. The inclusion of rhubarb introduces a unique flavor, and the use of almond butter and coconut adds richness.

- 1 cup ghee, melted
- ½ cup coconut cream, heated
- ¼ cup almond butter, soft
- ¼ tsp vanilla extract
- 2 tbsp. stevia
- juice and zest of 1 lemon
- ½ cup coconut, shredded

1. In blender, combine the ingredients and pulse well.
2. Pour mixture into round molds and freeze for 2 hours before serving.

PER SERVING

Calories: 141| Fat: 15g| Fiber: 1g| Carbs: 3g| Protein: 4 g

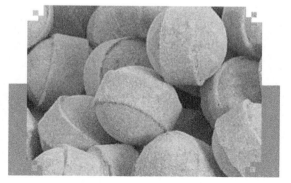

Keto Coffee with MCT Oil

Prep time: 5 minutes |Cook time: 5 minutes |Serves 1

Keto Coffee with MCT Oil is a suitable addition to an intermittent fasting eating plan. Designed for a ketogenic diet, it aligns with intermittent fasting by offering low carbohydrate content. Enriched with MCT oil, grass-fed butter or ghee, and heavy cream, it provides healthy fats that can promote satiety and sustained energy during the fasting window. The recipe is low in carbs, using sugar-free sweeteners, which aids in maintaining stable blood sugar levels and supporting ketosis during fasting. Its quick preparation makes it ideal for time-restricted eating, and you can customize the quantities of MCT oil, butter, cream, and sweetener to fit your preferences and calorie requirements. Enjoy it within your eating hours, being mindful of the added fats' calorie content.

- 1 cup of freshly brewed coffee
- 1-2 tablespoons of MCT oil (start with a lower amount if you're not used to it)
- 1-2 tablespoons of unsalted grass-fed butter or ghee
- 1-2 tablespoons of heavy cream (for added creaminess, adjust to your preference)
- A few drops of sugar-free sweetener (such as stevia or erythritol) to taste
- A pinch of ground cinnamon or cocoa powder for flavor

1. Brew a cup of your favorite coffee using your preferred method.
2. While the coffee is still hot, pour it into a blender or use an immersion blender.
3. Add 1-2 tablespoons of MCT oil to the coffee. MCT oil provides a quick source of energy and is a staple in keto coffee.
4. Add 1-2 tablespoons of unsalted grass-fed butter or ghee. This adds a creamy, rich texture and provides healthy fats.
5. Optionally, add 1-2 tablespoons of heavy cream if you like your coffee extra creamy. Adjust the amount to your taste.
6. If you prefer your coffee sweet, add a few drops of sugar-free sweetener. You can adjust the amount to suit your desired level of sweetness.
7. To enhance the flavor, you can sprinkle a pinch of ground cinnamon or cocoa powder into the coffee.
8. Blend all the ingredients together until the coffee becomes frothy and well-mixed.
9. Pour the blended keto coffee into your favorite mug and enjoy!

PER SERVING

Calories: 250| Fat: 25g| Fiber: 2g| Carbs: 3g| Protein: 1 g

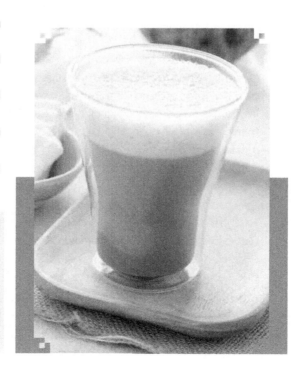

Strawberry Vanilla Smoothie

Prep time: 10 minutes | Cook time:5 minutes |Serves 1

The Strawberry Vanilla Smoothie, featuring ingredients like unsweetened almond milk, low-carb protein powder, frozen strawberries, heavy whipping cream, and MCT oil, can potentially be a suitable choice for individuals following an intermittent fasting eating plan. This smoothie offers a balance of protein, healthy fats, and minimal added sugars, making it a reasonable option for those looking to enjoy a delicious and filling treat during their eating window while maintaining control over calorie intake. The incorporation of fresh and frozen strawberries adds natural sweetness and flavor.

- 1 cup unsweetened vanilla-flavored or plain unsweetened almond milk
- 1 scoop sugar-free/low-carb protein powder (I use Quest Vanilla Milkshake flavor)
- 3 frozen strawberries
- 1 tablespoon heavy whipping cream
- 1 tablespoon MCT oil
- 4 to 6 ice cubes
- 1 fresh strawberry, for garnish (optional)

1. Place all the ingredients in a blender and blend until smooth.
2. If desired, slice a whole strawberry in half lengthwise, but not all the way through, and hang it from the rim of the glass.

PER SERVING

Calories: 292 | Fat: 22 g | Protein: 23 g | Total Carbs: 8 g

Berry Chia Pudding

Prep time: 10 minutes |Cook time: 20 minutes |Serves 1

Berry Chia Pudding, with its blend of fresh berries, chia seeds, coconut milk, and other ingredients, can be a suitable choice for individuals following an intermittent fasting eating plan. This pudding provides a balance of macronutrients, including protein, healthy fats, and dietary fiber, which can help promote a feeling of fullness and satisfaction during the eating window. The inclusion of whey protein powder and MCT oil can add extra nutritional benefits. The use of erythritol sweetener and sea salt enhances the flavor profile, aligning with the aim of making meals enjoyable within the eating window.

- ½ cup berries, fresh
- 8 tbsp. chia seeds
- 1 tbsp coconut flakes
- 1 tsp erythritol sweetener
- 2 tbsp. whey protein: powder
- 1/8 tsp sea salt
- 2 tbsp. MCT oil
- 3 cups coconut milk, unsweetened, full-fat

1. Place berries in a bowl, pour in milk, add oil and protein powder, sprinkle with salt and sweetener and blend using an immersion blender until smooth.
2. Place chia seeds in a serving bowl, top with berries mixture and stir well.
3. Refrigerate the pudding for a minimum of 4 hours, then garnish with coconut flakes and serve.

PER SERVING

Calories: 461.2 | Fat: 43 g | Protein: 6.7 g | Carb: 9 g | Fiber: 3 g

Slow Cooker Beef Bone Broth

Prep time: 15 minutes | Cook time:10 to 15 minutes |Serves 6 to 8

Slow Cooker Beef Bone Broth is a nutritious and versatile addition to an intermittent fasting eating plan. This broth, made from pastured beef bones, celery, onion, garlic, and spices, is a great source of essential nutrients, including collagen and minerals. Consuming bone broth during the eating window can provide a feeling of satiety, helping individuals stay on track with their fasting goals. The low-calorie nature of the broth makes it an ideal choice for those aiming to manage calorie intake while enjoying a nutrient-rich food. The addition of apple cider vinegar and seasoning with pink Himalayan salt and black pepper enhances the flavor profile and aligns with the goal of making meals enjoyable during the eating window. This slow cooker beef bone broth can be a valuable component of an intermittent fasting regimen, whether consumed on its own or as a base for various dishes, while being mindful of overall caloric consumption.

- 3 to 4 pounds pastured beef bones
- 3 stalks celery, quartered
- 1 large yellow onion, quartered
- 4 cloves garlic, smashed with the side of a knife
- 2 tablespoons apple cider vinegar
- 3 bay leaves
- 1 tablespoon black peppercorns
- Filtered water
- Pink Himalayan salt and ground black pepper

1. Place the bones, celery, onion, garlic, vinegar, bay leaves, and peppercorns in a 6-quart or larger slow cooker. Fill the slow cooker about two-thirds full with filtered water, just enough to submerge the bones.
2. Cover and make sure the slow cooker is in a safe spot on the counter, not too close to the edge and not touching any other items. Cook on low for 10
3. to 15 hours. (I often let my broth simmer overnight.) During cooking, add more water if needed to keep the bones submerged.
4. Use tongs to remove the bones and large vegetable pieces. Strain the broth through a fine-mesh strainer. Season with salt and pepper to taste.
5. Store the broth in an airtight container in the refrigerator for up to 5
6. days or in the freezer for up to several months.

PER SERVING

Calories: 65 | Fat: 4 g | Protein: 6 g | Total Carbs: 2 g

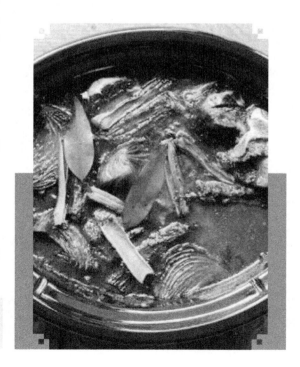

Coffee Shake

Prep time: 5 minutes | Cook time:5 minutes |Serves 1

The Coffee Shake recipe is an option for an intermittent fasting eating plan, especially for those following a ketogenic diet due to its low carbohydrate content. It features full-fat coconut milk, which provides healthy fats for satiety, aligning well with fasting principles. The use of erythritol or liquid stevia as sweeteners, coupled with cocoa powder and instant coffee granules, keeps the shake low in carbs, promoting stable blood sugar levels during fasting. With its quick preparation, it's a convenient choice for time-restricted eating, suitable for breakfast or a snack within your eating window. You can also customize the level of sweetness and the type of sweetener to match your preferences and calorie requirements. To ensure it suits your intermittent fasting plan, consume it within your designated eating hours and be mindful of the calorie content from fats and sweeteners.

- 1 cup (240 ml) full-fat coconut milk
- ½ cup (120 ml) water
- 4 ice cubes
- 2 tablespoons coconut oil, unflavored MCT oil powder, or ghee
- 1½ tablespoons cocoa powder
- 1½ teaspoons erythritol, or 2 drops liquid stevia
- ½ teaspoon instant coffee granules

1. Place all the ingredients in a blender or food processor. Blend on high until the ice is broken up completely and the texture of the shake is smooth.
2. Transfer to a 14-ounce (415-ml) or larger glass. Best enjoyed immediately.

PER SERVING

Calories: 757 | Total Fat: 76 g |Carbs: 12.3 g | Fiber: 2.7 g | Protein: 6.1 g

Chocolate Avocado Pudding

Prep time: 5 minutes | Cook time:5 minutes |Serves 2

Chocolate Avocado Pudding can be a suitable dessert option for individuals following an intermittent fasting eating plan. This pudding is a balanced choice, with ingredients like avocado, heavy whipping cream, and cocoa powder, offering a combination of healthy fats and flavor. The use of Swerve confectioners' sweetener aligns with low-carb and keto-friendly dietary goals. Vanilla extract enhances the taste of the pudding. While this dessert can be a part of an intermittent fasting regimen, it should be consumed mindfully and balanced with other nutrient-rich foods to align with your daily dietary objectives. The optional addition of Keto Whipped Cream can enhance the experience while still being mindful of calorie intake during the eating window.

- 1 avocado, soft but not super ripe, halved and pitted
- 2 tablespoons heavy whipping cream
- 2 tablespoons Swerve confectioners'-style sweetener
- 1 heaping tablespoon unsweetened cocoa powder
- ½ teaspoon vanilla extract
- Keto Whipped Cream, for topping (optional)

1. Scoop the flesh of the avocado into a bowl. Add the rest of the ingredients and blend with a hand mixer until smooth. Place in the refrigerator to chill for 30 minutes.
2. Serve topped with fresh whipped cream, if desired.

PER SERVING

Calories: 175 | Fat: 16 g | Protein: 2 g | Total Carbs: 16 g

Slow Cooker Loaded Cauliflower Soup

Prep time: 15 minutes | Cook time: 4 or 8 hours |Serves 10

Slow Cooker Loaded Cauliflower Soup can be a satisfying choice for individuals following an intermittent fasting eating plan. This hearty soup, made with cauliflower, chicken broth, cheese, and bacon, offers a combination of protein, healthy fats, and dietary fiber, which can contribute to a sense of fullness and enjoyment during the eating window. The inclusion of heavy whipping cream and butter adds richness and flavor to the soup. Seasoning with salt and pepper enhances the taste, aligning with the aim of making meals pleasant within the eating window.

- 10 slices bacon
- 2 large or 3 small heads cauliflower
- 4 cups chicken broth
- ½ large yellow onion, chopped (about 1⅓ cups)
- 3 cloves garlic, pressed
- ¼ cup (½ stick) salted butter
- 2 cups shredded cheddar cheese, plus extra for garnish
- 1 cup heavy whipping cream
- Salt and pepper
- Snipped fresh chives or sliced green onions, for garnish (optional)

1. Fry the bacon in a large skillet over medium heat. Transfer to a paper towel–lined plate, allow to cool, and then chop. Set aside in the refrigerator.
2. Core the heads of cauliflower and cut the cauliflower into florets.
3. Place the florets in a food processor and chop into small to medium-sized pieces. (Don't rice it.)
4. In a large slow cooker (I use a 5½-quart slow cooker), combine the chicken broth, onion, garlic, butter, and cauliflower. Stir, cover, and cook on high for 4 hours or on low for 8 hours.
5. Once the cauliflower is tender, switch the slow cooker to the keep warm setting and use a whisk to stir and mash the cauliflower to a smooth
6. consistency.
7. Add about three-quarters of the chopped bacon, the cheese, and the cream. Season with salt and pepper to taste. Stir well until the cheese is melted.
8. Serve garnished with additional cheese, the remaining bacon, and chives or green onions, if desired.

PER SERVING

Calories: 282 | Fat: 22 g | Protein: 12 g | Total Carbs: 8 g

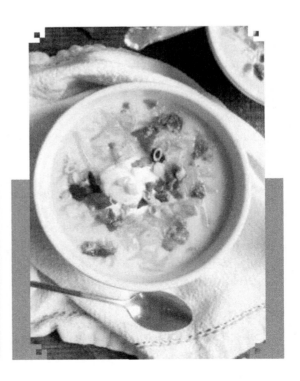

Peanut Butter Bars

Prep time: 10 minutes |Cook time: 20 minutes |Serves 6

Peanut Butter Bars can be a convenient option for those adhering to an intermittent fasting eating plan, particularly if you're looking for a satisfying and indulgent treat within your eating window. These bars are made with ground almond flour, peanut butter, and erythritol sweetener, providing a source of fats and a touch of sweetness. The chocolate coating enhances the flavor while maintaining a low-carb approach, which can align with intermittent fasting goals. Enjoying these peanut butter bars as an occasional treat can make the fasting experience more enjoyable while still adhering to the plan's guidelines.

- 5 tbsp. ground almond flour
- 1 tsp vanilla extract, unsweetened
- ½ cup peanut butter, unsweetened
- 4 tbsp. erythritol sweetener
- 4 tbsp. butter, unsalted, melted
- 2.5 oz. chocolate, sugar-free

1. Place all filling ingredients in a bowl and stir well until smooth.
2. Take a rectangular molds silicone tray, add the prepared mixture in it and freeze for 30 minutes or until firm.
3. Then place chocolate into a heatproof bowl and microwave for 2 minutes or until chocolate has melted.
4. Pour the melted chocolate evenly on frozen bars, about 0.2-inch thick, and continue freezing the bars until solid, saving the remaining melted chocolate.
5. Return the bars into the freezer until chilled and solid and then serve.

PER SERVING

Calories: 315 | Fat: 27.3 g | Protein: 9.7 g | Net Carb: 5 g | Fiber: 1.5 g

Coconut and Almond Chocolate Bars

Prep time: 10 minutes |Cook time: 20 minutes |Serves 15

Coconut and Almond Chocolate Bars are a suitable treat for individuals following an intermittent fasting eating plan, particularly when they aim to indulge in a satisfying dessert during their eating window. These bars combine the richness of dark chocolate with sliced almonds, coconut flakes, and chia seeds. The almonds provide healthy fats and protein, while the coconut oil and flakes add a delightful tropical flavor. By using dark chocolate and minimal added sugar, these bars align with low-carb and low-sugar dietary preferences common in many fasting regimens.

- 3.5 oz. dark chocolate, unsweetened
- 1 1/2 cups sliced almond
- 1 tbsp chia seeds
- 1 cup coconut flakes
- 1/4 tsp sea salt
- 3/4 cup coconut oil, melted
- 4 tbsp. chopped almonds

1. Preheat oven to 350 F.
2. Meanwhile, place a skillet over medium heat, add coconut flakes and cook for 5 minutes or until toasted. Set aside.
3. Meanwhile, melt chocolate in microwave for 2 minutes.
4. Drizzle chocolate over frozen almond-coconut mixture, then sprinkle with chopped almonds and continue freezing for 5 minutes.
5. Then cut into squares and serve.

PER SERVING

Calories: 227 | Fat: 22.6 g | Protein: 2.7 g | Net Carb: 2.8 g | Fiber: 2.6 g

Low Carb Recipes

Creamy Turkey and Bell Pepper Casserole

Prep time: 5 minutes | Cook time: 30 minutes |Serves 5

The Creamy Turkey and Bell Pepper Casserole can be a favorable option for those following an intermittent fasting eating plan. It provides a substantial and satisfying meal during the eating window. This casserole combines turkey, bell peppers, and a creamy sauce enriched with double cream and Swiss cheese, offering a mix of protein, healthy fats, and flavor. The inclusion of turkey as the primary protein source makes it a lean and nutritious choice, while the bell peppers add a touch of freshness and vitamins. The creamy sauce contributes richness, making the meal enjoyable while adhering to fasting guidelines. However, it's important to be mindful of portion size and calorie intake, especially if you're following a specific fasting protocol with caloric restrictions during the eating period. Overall, this casserole can be a tasty and filling addition to your intermittent fasting meal plan.

- 3 teaspoons olive oil
- 1 cup bell peppers, sliced
- 1 yellow onion, thinly sliced
- 1 ½ pounds turkey breast
- Se salt and ground black pepper, to taste
- 1 cup chicken bone broth
- 1 cup double cream
- 1/2 cup Swiss cheese, shredded

1. Heat 2 teaspoons of the olive oil in a sauté pan over a moderate flame. Sauté the peppers and onion until they have softened; reserve.
2. In the same sauté pan, heat the remaining teaspoon of olive oil and sear the turkey breasts until no longer pink.
3. Layer the peppers and onions in a lightly greased baking pan. Add the turkey breast; sprinkle with salt and pepper.
4. Mix the chicken bone broth with the double cream; pour the mixture over the turkey breasts. Bake in the preheated oven at 350 degrees F for 20 minutes; top with the Swiss cheese.
5. Bake an additional 5 minutes or until golden brown on top. Bon appétit!

PER SERVING

Calories: 464 | Fat: 28.5g | Carbs: 4.5g | Protein: 45.4g | Fiber: 0.3g

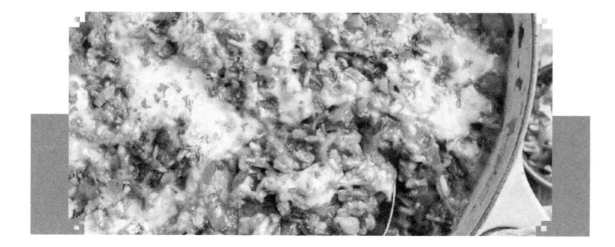

Easy and Tender Pork Cutlets

Prep time: 5 minutes | Cook time: 15 minutes |Serves 4

These Easy and Tender Pork Cutlets are a convenient and quick option for an intermittent fasting eating plan. They provide a source of protein with the pork cutlets, and the cream of onion soup adds flavor and richness to the dish. This meal is prepared in a relatively short amount of time, which can be beneficial during the eating window in an intermittent fasting regimen, making it easy to have a satisfying and tasty meal without an extended preparation period. However, when incorporating this dish into your fasting plan, it's essential to pay attention to portion sizes and ingredients to ensure they align with your fasting goals and dietary preferences.

- 2 tablespoons olive oil
- 4 pork cutlets
- 1/4 cup cream of onion soup
- 1/2 teaspoon paprika
- Sea salt and ground black pepper, to taste

1. Heat the olive oil in a sauté pan over moderate heat. Once hot, sear the pork cutlets for 5 to 6 minutes, turning once or twice to ensure even cooking.
2. Add in the cream of onion soup, paprika, salt, and black pepper. Cook for a further 3 minutes until heated through. The meat thermometer should register 145 degrees F.
3. Serve in individual plates garnished with freshly snipped chives if desired. Enjoy!

PER SERVING

Calories: 395 | Fat: 24.4g | Carbs: 0.8g | Protein: 40.3g | Fiber:0.1g

Grilled Beef Short Loin

Prep time: 5 minutes | Cook time:30 minutes | Servin 3

Grilled Beef Short Loin is a protein-rich option suitable for an intermittent fasting eating plan. This dish provides a good source of beef short loin, seasoned with herbs like thyme and rosemary, as well as garlic powder, which enhances the flavor. It's relatively easy to prepare, which is practical for those adhering to intermittent fasting and seeking a straightforward, satisfying meal during their eating window. The lean protein content can help maintain satiety, making it an excellent choice for those following a fasting regimen.

- 1 ½ pounds beef short loin
- 2 thyme sprigs, chopped
- 1 rosemary sprig, chopped
- 1 teaspoon garlic powder
- Sea salt and ground black pepper, to taste

1. Place all of the above ingredients in a re-sealable zipper bag. Shake until the beef short loin is well coated on all sides.
2. Cook on a preheated grill for 15 to 20 minutes, flipping once or twice during the cooking time.
3. Let it stand for 5 minutes before slicing and serving. Bon appétit!

PER SERVING

Calories: 313| Fat: 11.6g | Carbs: 0.1g | Protein: 52g | Fiber: 0.1g

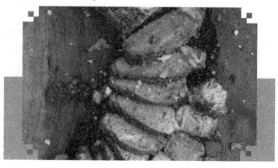

Haddock Fillets with Mediterranean Sauce

Prep time: 5 minutes | Cook time: 30 minutes |Serves 4

Haddock Fillets with Mediterranean Sauce is a nutritious option for individuals following an intermittent fasting eating plan. Haddock is a lean protein source that complements fasting goals by providing satiety without excess calories. The Mediterranean sauce, made from ingredients like scallions, dill, oregano, basil, mayonnaise, and cream cheese, enhances the flavor of the dish while keeping it low in carbohydrates, suitable for fasting periods. This meal is easy to prepare and can be enjoyed during your eating window, providing a flavorful and protein-rich option to help you feel satisfied.

- 1 pound haddock fillets
- 1 tablespoon olive oil
- Sea salt and freshly cracked black pepper, to taste Mediterranean Sauce:
- 2 scallions, chopped
- 1/2 teaspoon dill weed
- 1/2 teaspoon oregano
- 1 teaspoon basil
- 1/4 cup mayonnaise
- 1/4 cup cream cheese, at room temperature

1. Start by preheating your oven to 360 degrees F. Toss the haddock fillets with the olive oil, salt, and black pepper.
2. Cover with foil and bake for 20 to 25 minutes.
3. In the meantime, make the sauce by whisking all ingredients until well combined. Serve with the warm haddock fillets and enjoy!

PER SERVING

Calories: 260 | Fat: 19.1g | Carbs: 1.3g | Protein: 19.6g | Fiber: 0.3g

Paprika Omelet with Goat Cheese

Prep time: 5 minutes | Cook time: 10 minutes |Serves 2

The Paprika Omelet with Goat Cheese is a great option for those on an intermittent fasting eating plan. This meal is packed with healthy fats and protein, which can help keep you satiated during your fasting window. Eggs provide essential nutrients and protein, while goat cheese adds a creamy texture and rich flavor without many carbohydrates. The quick and straightforward preparation of this dish makes it suitable for a busy fasting schedule.

- 2 teaspoons ghee, room temperature
- 4 eggs, whisked
- 4 tablespoons goat cheese
- 1 teaspoon paprika
- Sea salt and ground black pepper, to taste

1. Melt the ghee in a pan over medium heat.
2. Add the whisked eggs to the pan and cover with the lid; reduce the heat to medium-low.
3. Cook for 4 minutes; now, stir in the cheese and paprika; continue to cook an additional 3 minutes or until cheese has melted.
4. Season with salt and pepper and serve immediately. Enjoy!

PER SERVING

Calories: 287 | Fat: 22.6g | Carbs: 1.3g | Fiber: 0g | Protein: 19.8g

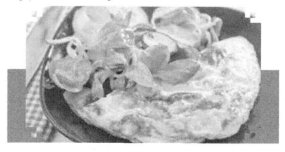

Vegetarian Recipes

Creamy Broccoli Casserole

Prep Time: 15 Minutes | Cook Time: 6 Hours | Serves 6

The Creamy Broccoli Casserole is a suitable choice for individuals following an intermittent fasting eating plan. This recipe provides a balanced mix of vegetables, fats, and protein. The broccoli and cauliflower contribute to fiber intake, which can help maintain satiety during fasting periods.The inclusion of almond flour and coconut milk offers healthy fats, making this dish suitable for those practicing intermittent fasting, as fats can help sustain energy levels. The use of nutmeg and gouda cheese adds a flavorful touch to the casserole. When incorporating this casserole into your eating window, it can serve as a hearty and nutritious meal, contributing to your daily nutrient needs and helping you feel full.

- 1 tablespoon extra-virgin olive oil
- 1 pound broccoli, cut into florets
- 1 pound cauliflower, cut into florets
- ¼ cup almond flour
- 2 cups coconut milk
- ½ teaspoon ground nutmeg
- pinch freshly ground black pepper
- 1½ cups shredded gouda cheese, divided

1. Lightly grease the insert of the slow cooker with the olive oil.
2. Place the broccoli and cauliflower in the insert.
3. In a small bowl, stir together the almond flour, coconut milk, nutmeg, pepper, and 1 cup of the cheese.
4. Pour the coconut milk mixture over the vegetables and top the casserole with the remaining ½ cup of the cheese.
5. Cover and cook on low for 6 hours.
6. Serve warm.

PER SERVING:

Calories: 377|Total Fat: 32g|Protein: 16g|Total Carbs: 12g|Fiber: 6g

Greek Cottage Cheese Salad

Prep time: 5 minutes | Cook time:5 minutes |Serves 1

The Greek Cottage Cheese Salad is a nutritious option for individuals following an intermittent fasting eating plan. This salad combines cottage cheese, cherry tomatoes, scallions, cucumber, olive oil, and Kalamata olives, offering a variety of flavors and textures. Cottage cheese provides a good source of and satisfied during your eating window. The addition of fresh vegetables like cherry tomatoes, scallions, and cucumber contributes essential vitamins and minerals. Olive oil offers healthy fats and adds a Mediterranean flavor to the salad.This salad can serve as a satisfying meal or a side dish, depending on your fasting goals and portion size. It's a balanced option that can fit well into your eating window during intermittent fasting.

- 1 cup 4-percent cottage cheese
- ⅓ cup halved cherry tomatoes
- 1 tablespoon chopped scallion, white part only
- ⅓ cup peeled and diced cucumber
- 2 tablespoons olive oil
- ½ cup Kalamata olives
- Salt
- Freshly ground black pepper

1. In a serving bowl, mix together the cottage cheese, cherry tomatoes, scallion, cucumber, olive oil, and olives, and season with salt and pepper as needed.

PER SERVING

Calories: 610 | Fat: 51g | Protein: 27g | Total Carbs: 15g | Fiber: 4g |Protein: 19% | Carbs: 9%

Broccoli Stir-Fry

Prep time: 5 minutes | Cook time:10 minutes |Serves 1

The Broccoli Stir-Fry is a balanced meal option suitable for individuals practicing intermittent fasting. This stir-fry combines nutrient-rich ingredients to create a satisfying dish for your eating window. Fresh spinach provides essential vitamins and minerals while adding a vibrant green color to your plate. Broccoli and cauliflower rice offer fiber and cruciferous vegetable goodness, and seitan strips contribute plant-based protein.The sesame oil and soy sauce dressing infuses the dish with a savory and umami flavor. Avocado slices add a creamy and satisfying element to the meal, thanks to their healthy fats.Overall, this Broccoli Stir-Fry is a filling and nutritious choice for your eating window during intermittent fasting.

- 1 cup fresh spinach
- 1 tablespoon coconut oil
- ½ cup broccoli florets
- 1 cup frozen cauliflower rice
- 2 ounces seitan strips or cubes
- 1 tablespoon toasted sesame oil
- 1 tablespoon soy sauce
- ½ avocado, sliced

1. In a dry, nonstick pan over medium heat, wilt the spinach leaves. Remove from the heat and transfer to a serving plate.
2. Turn the temperature up to medium high, and in the same skillet, melt the coconut oil. Add the broccoli and frozen cauliflower rice. Cook for 5 to 6 minutes or until tender.
3. Place the vegetables on the wilted spinach. Top with the seitan.
4. In a small bowl, mix together the sesame oil and soy sauce.
5. Pour the dressing over the seitan and vegetables. Top with the avocado slices and enjoy warm.

PER SERVING

Calories: 664 | Fat: 44g | Protein: 49g | Total Carbs: 18g | Fiber: 13g

Avocado Pesto Panini

Prep time: 5 minutes | Cook time:10 minutes |Serves 1

The Avocado Pesto Panini is a delightful and wholesome sandwich option for individuals practicing intermittent fasting. It combines quality ingredients to create a balanced and satisfying meal during your eating window.Sliced avocado adds a creamy texture and healthy fats to the panini, making it even more satisfying. When grilled on the griddle, the bread becomes golden and crispy, enhancing the overall texture of the sandwich.This Avocado Pesto Panini is an excellent choice to enjoy during your eating window while intermittent fasting.

- 2 tablespoons grass-fed butter, at room temperature
- 2 slices Easy Keto Bread or store bought
- 1 tablespoon basil pesto
- 2 slices Gruyère cheese
- ½ medium avocado, sliced

1. Heat a small griddle over medium heat.
2. Spread the butter on one side of each slice of bread.
3. Place one piece of bread, butter-side down, on the griddle and then layer the pesto, cheese, and avocado on top.
4. Allow to cook for 4 to 5 minutes; then flip carefully and cook for an additional 3 to 4 minutes, or until the bread is golden brown.

PER SERVING

Calories: 824 | Fat: 72g | Protein: 29g | Total Carbs: 15g | Fiber: 8g

Classic Creamy Coleslaw

Prep time: 5 minutes | Cook time:5 minutes |Serves 1

The Classic Creamy Coleslaw is a quick and easy recipe suitable for a single serving. This coleslaw is both vegan-friendly and low in carbohydrates, making it a suitable choice for various dietary preferences. The creamy coleslaw dressing is created using veganaise, a vegan alternative to traditional mayonnaise. To add a tangy and slightly sweet flavor to the dressing, white vinegar and a few drops of liquid stevia are included. Dry mustard, salt, and freshly ground black pepper further enhance the taste.The prepared coleslaw mix simplifies the process, allowing you to enjoy the classic coleslaw combination of shredded cabbage and carrots without the need for extensive chopping or grating.To provide a source of plant-based protein, seitan strips are added to the coleslaw. Seitan, often known as wheat meat, has a chewy and meat-like texture, making it a satisfying addition to the dish.This single-serving Classic Creamy Coleslaw offers a balance of creamy, tangy, and slightly sweet flavors, perfect for those looking for a light and satisfying meal.

- 3 tablespoons veganaise
- ½ tablespoon white vinegar
- 3 drops liquid stevia
- ¼ teaspoon dry mustard
- ¼ teaspoon salt
- ¼ teaspoon freshly ground black pepper
- 1 cup prepared coleslaw mix
- 3½ ounces seitan strips

1. In a small bowl, stir together the veganaise, vinegar, stevia, mustard, salt, and pepper until well combined.
2. Add the coleslaw mix and fold it in gently.
3. Top with the seitan and add more pepper, if needed.

PER SERVING

Calories: 381 | Fat: 29g | Protein: 22g | Total Carbs: 8g | Fiber: 3g

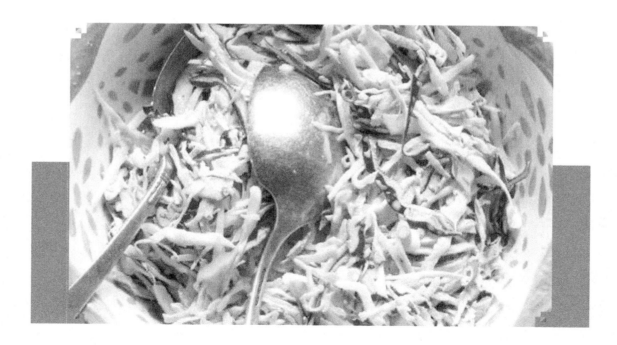

Chapter 10

4-Week Meal Plan

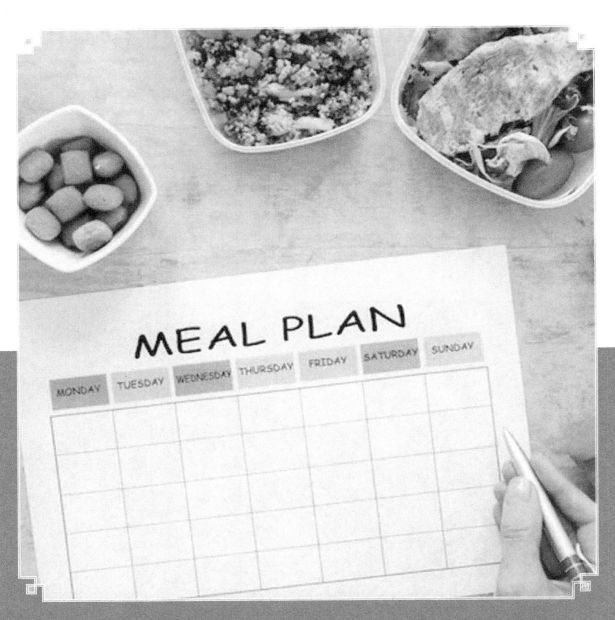

24-Hour Fasting Protocol

In this particular fasting regimen, you will abstain from food for a full 24-hour period, either from lunch one day to lunch the next day or from dinner one day to dinner the next day, three times a week. Additionally, it involves a daily 16-hour fast, which essentially means skipping breakfast and eating within an eight-hour window on non-fasting days. We've observed that this fasting pattern is effective for gradual weight loss in our Intensive Dietary Management Program. However, for those who prefer a less rigorous approach, you can opt for just two 24-hour fasts per week.

On days when you're allowed to eat, we recommend a diet that is low in refined carbohydrates and rich in natural fats. Strive to consume whole, unprocessed foods while minimizing your intake of processed or pre-packaged foods. This fasting protocol allows for a daily meal, making it suitable for individuals who require medication with food or have busy schedules. For instance, dinner can still serve as a time for family connection, as you'll have that opportunity on this fasting schedule. This type of fasting routine also conveniently aligns with a typical work schedule.

As an example, consider fasting from dinner on Sunday evening until dinner on Monday evening. If you finish your Sunday dinner at 7:30 p.m., you would not have your next dinner until 7:30 p.m. on Monday. The suggested meals are designed to support a low-carb, high-healthy-fat diet.

SUNDAY

Breakfast: FAST
Break your fast:
Lunch: Full Meal Deal
Dinner: Cream Cheese Pancakes

MONDAY

Breakfast: FAST
Lunch: FAST
Break your fast:
Dinner: Bacon-Wrapped Avocado Fries

TUESDAY

Breakfast: FAST
Lunch: Cabbage & Sausage with Bacon
Dinner: Rhubarb Bombs

WEDNESDAY

Breakfast: FAST
Lunch: FAST
Break your fast:
Dinner: Peanut Butter Bars

THURSDAY

Breakfast: FAST
Break your fast:
Lunch: Cheesy Broccoli
Dinner: Keto Chocolate Frosty

FRIDAY

Breakfast: FAST
Lunch: FAST
Break your fast:
Dinner: Chocolate Avocado Pudding

SATURDAY

Breakfast: FAST
Break your fast:
Lunch: Cream Cheese Pancakes
Dinner: Full Meal Deal

Sample of a three-times-per-week 24-hour fasting regimen. This shows fasting from dinner to dinner, but you could also fast from lunch to lunch.

36-Hour Fasting Protocol

In this thirty-six-hour fasting plan, you'll abstain from food for the entire day on at least three days each week. Unlike the twenty-four-hour fasting protocol, fasting days do not include any meals; you only consume fasting fluids. This approach is generally more effective for weight loss compared to the twenty-four-hour fasting protocol, and the extended fasting period is particularly beneficial for lowering blood sugar levels, making it a potential choice for those with prediabetes. Additionally, some individuals find the simplicity of fasting for the entire day on fasting days preferable to the one-meal approach in the twenty-four-hour protocol.

On days when you are allowed to eat, we recommend a diet that is low in refined carbohydrates and rich in natural fats. Strive to consume whole, unprocessed foods while minimizing your intake of processed or prepared foods as much as possible.

As an example, consider fasting from dinner on Sunday night until breakfast on Tuesday morning. If you finish dinner on Sunday at 7:30 p.m., you would not eat again until breakfast on Tuesday morning at 7:30 a.m. On non-fasting days, you can have breakfast, lunch, and dinner as usual.

SUNDAY

Breakfast: Cream Cheese Pancakes
Lunch: Full Meal Deal
Dinner: Cheesy Broccoli

MONDAY

Breakfast: FAST
Lunch: FAST
Dinner: FAST

TUESDAY

Breakfast: Cabbage & Sausage with Bacon
Lunch: Coconut Curry and Ginger Chicken Meatballs
Dinner: Berry Chia Pudding

WEDNESDAY

Breakfast: FAST
Lunch: FAST
Dinner: FAST

THURSDAY

Breakfast: Cabbage & Sausage with Bacon
Lunch: Coconut Curry and Ginger Chicken Meatballs
Dinner: Chocolate Avocado Pudding

FRIDAY

Breakfast: FAST
Lunch: FAST
Dinner: FAST

SATURDAY

Breakfast: Cream Cheese Pancakes
Lunch: Full Meal Deal
Dinner: Cheesy Broccoli

Sample of a three-times-per-week 36-hour fasting regimen. No meals or snacks of any kind are consumed on the fasting days, but you may consume any fasting fluid.

42-Hour Fasting Protocol

In this forty-two-hour fasting plan, you will fast for the entire day on at least three days each week, and you'll also skip breakfast every day, whether it's a fasting day or not. On fasting days, your intake is restricted to fasting fluids.

In our Intensive Dietary Management Program, we primarily utilize this forty-two-hour fasting protocol for managing type

2 diabetes. The prolonged fasting period provides more time for blood glucose and insulin levels to decrease. However, if you are taking medications, it's crucial to consult your physician before starting this fasting regimen to prevent the risk of low blood sugar. While we expect and aim for blood sugar levels to decrease, excessive medication might lead to dangerously low levels, necessitating the consumption of sugar to raise it, which contradicts the purpose of fasting.

On days when you can eat, we recommend a diet that is low in refined carbohydrates and rich in natural fats. It's important to focus on consuming whole, unprocessed foods and minimizing your intake of processed or prepared foods as much as possible.

As an example, consider fasting from dinner on Sunday night until lunch on Tuesday. If you finish dinner on Sunday at 7:30 p.m., you would not resume eating until lunch on Tuesday afternoon at 1:30 p.m. On non-fasting days, you should have lunch and dinner, but breakfast is skipped.

SUNDAY

Breakfast: FAST
Lunch: Easy and Tender Pork Cutlets
Dinner: Broccoli Stir-Fry

MONDAY

Breakfast: FAST
Lunch: FAST
Dinner: FAST

TUESDAY

Breakfast: FAST
Lunch: Haddock Fillets with Mediterranean Sauce
Dinner: Classic Creamy Coleslaw

WEDNESDAY

Breakfast: FAST
Lunch: FAST
Dinner: FAST

THURSDAY

Breakfast: FAST
Lunch: Grilled Beef Short Loin
Dinner: Greek Cottage Cheese Salad

FRIDAY

Breakfast: FAST
Lunch: FAST
Dinner: FAST

SATURDAY

Breakfast: FAST
Lunch: Paprika Omelet with Goat Cheese
Dinner: Avocado Pesto Panini

Sample of a three-times-per-week 42-hour fasting regimen. No meals or snacks of any kind are consumed on the fasting days, but you may consume any fasting fluid. Breakfast is not consumed on nonfasting or fasting days.

7- To 14-Day Fasting Protocol

This fasting protocol entails an extended fast lasting from seven to fourteen consecutive days, which means going without meals or snacks for a continuous period of seven to fourteen days. During the fasting period, you are restricted to consuming fasting fluids only.

In our Intensive Dietary Management Program, we typically employ this protocol for severe cases of diabetes or morbid obesity. In situations where prompt management of diabetes and obesity is imperative, we may recommend commencing therapy with this protocol and then transitioning to a forty-two-hour fasting regimen. It's also a useful approach when dealing with weight loss plateaus or following periods of weight regain, such as holiday seasons and vacations (e.g., cruises). Knowing that you have this protocol to follow after a period of celebration can provide you with the freedom to enjoy without guilt.

It's crucial to emphasize that this is an extremely intensive regimen and should only be undertaken under the supervision of a healthcare professional. If you are taking medications, adjustments may be necessary before starting the fast. As part of this protocol, we recommend daily use of a general multivitamin to prevent micronutrient deficiencies, and your physician may want to monitor your bloodwork throughout the fast.

It's important to note that hunger does not continually worsen during the fast. Day 2 is typically the most challenging day, as studies on the hunger hormone ghrelin indicate that it peaks on the second day of extended fasting and then gradually decreases. Generally, each day becomes more manageable, and many individuals report after seven days that they feel they could have continued fasting indefinitely.

Due to the risk of refeeding syndrome, we do not typically extend the fasting period beyond fourteen days. Instead, we recommend using an alternate-day fasting schedule such as the thirty-six-hour or forty-two-hour protocol before repeating the seven- to fourteen-day fast. We advise undertaking seven-day fasts no more than once a month and fourteen-day fasts no more than every six weeks.

Importantly, if at any point during the fast you do not feel well, for any reason, it is crucial to stop the fast.

Under this protocol, you will abstain from meals or snacks for at least seven full days, beginning, for instance, on a Sunday morning and continuing through Saturday night.

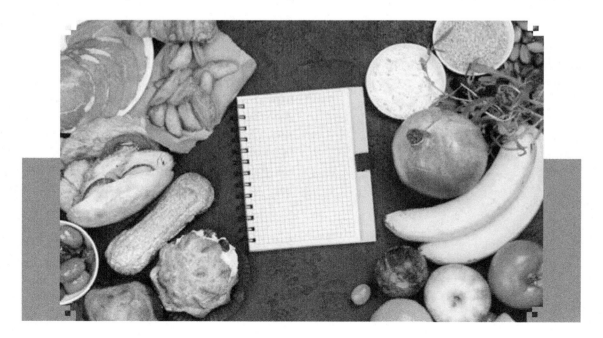

Conclusion

In this "She is Fasting" book you have experienced a remarkable journey. It has pulled you through courage, domination, and incredible resilience. In this journey, you have learned more about your body. In this book, I have also exposed many methods that are harmful for you yet we have been following them for ages. And most importantly the one-size-fits-all approaches are shattered by our options of fasting.

From the very first of this book, I helped you to understand the concept of "She is Fasting" is not an insult but a matter of pride. Just like men and women have many differences, women have many unique features of themselves as well. For that reason, it is impossible to gain permanent results from other types of one-size-fits-all approaches. For that reason, I designed this book according to women's problems and solutions to them.

Fasting is a lifesaver for all those women who are suffering from hormonal problems. It effectively deals with the most common problems women face like weight gain, brain fog, tiredness, blood sugar, and many more. Fasting does all of these without strict diets, intense workout plans, and hormone replacement therapy. This not only balances your hormones but also lowers the risk of age-related problems by maintaining muscle mass.

The fact that makes fasting the best plan is its flexibility. It has no strict rules and there are a variety of fasts you can practice. For that reason, you can practice it without sparing any extra time for it. A fun fact about fasting is every fasting method targets some special hormones. In simple words, you have to fast according to your goals. Women suffering from PCOS and other hormone-related disorders are most benefited from different types of fast I have included in this book.

Another important thing about fasting that I have told you before is that the fasting cycle should match your menopausal cycle. For that reason, I have included the most common 3 types of fasting cycles and created your fasting routine according to them. Everything you need to know about fasting is included in this "She is Fasting" book. I have also included how you can make fasting effortless with some easy hacks. If you follow the fasting routine, you do not have to worry about anything. And last but not least I have included recipes that will help you in your fasting journey. These recipes are according to our fast targets so you have to determine which one goes perfectly with your condition.

This book is not only a fasting plan and a lot of information about fasting but this is my years of experience and research in one book. It took me a long time to research all these theories and create a perfect fasting book for all the women around the world. I want all of the girls to live a healthy life and feel like a teenager again. So read this book and try everything I have included.

I assure you that fasting according to this book will change your life and you will see your body differently from now. It will help you live a healthy life and make you feel younger than ever. Please share this book with your friends, family, and loved ones to encourage them to live a healthy life.

Dr Teresa Hill

Printed in Great Britain
by Amazon